Keto Chaffle Recipes Cookbook

Sensational Keto Chaffle Recipes to Lose Weight with Flavor

Karla Dejacono

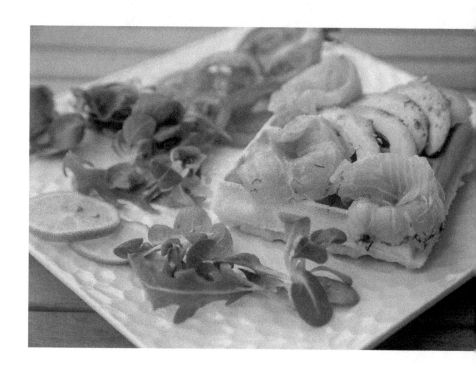

TABLE OF CONTENT

4

any policies, processes, or Directions: contained within is the solitary and utter responsibility of the recipient reader. Under no circumstances will any legal responsibility or blame be held against the publisher for any reparation, damages, or monetary loss due to the information herein, either directly or indirectly.

Respective authors own all copyrights not held by the publisher.

The information herein is offered for informational purposes solely, and is universal as so. The presentation of the information is without contract or any type of guarantee assurance.

The trademarks that are used are without any consent, and the publication of the trademark is without permission or backing by the trademark owner. All trademarks and brands within this book are for clarifying purposes only and are the owned by the owners themselves, not affiliated with this document.

LUNCH AND DINNER CHAFFLES

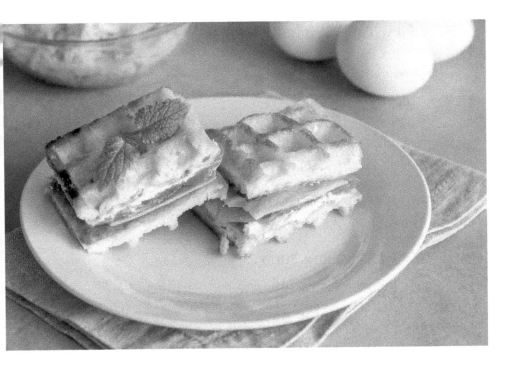

1. Garlic And Spinach chaffles

Servings: 2

Cooking Time:5 minutes

Ingredients:

- 1 cup egg whites .
- 1 tsp Italian spice
- 2 tsps. coconut flour
- 1/2 tsp vanilla
- 1 tsp baking powder
- 1 tsp baking soda
- 1 cup mozzarella cheese, grated
- 1/2 tsp garlic powder
- 1 cup chopped spinach

Directions:

1. switch on your square waffle maker. Spray with non-stick spray.
2. Beat egg whites with beater, until fluffy and white.
3. Add pumpkin puree, pumpkin pie spice, coconut flour in egg whites and beat again.
4. Stir in the cheese, powder, garlic powder, baking soda, and powder.
5. Sprinkle chopped spinach on a warm maker

6. Pour the batter in waffle maker over chopped spinach
7. Close the maker and cook for about 4-5 minutes.
8. Remove chaffles from the maker.
9. Serve hot and enjoy!

Nutritional Values: Per Servings: Protein: 52 % 88kcal Fat: 41% 69 kcal Carbohydrates: 7% 12 kcal

2. Chaffle Sandwich

Servings: 2

Cooking Time: 8 Minutes

Ingredients:

Chaffle bread

- 1/2 cup mozzarella cheese, shredded
- 1 egg
- 1 tbs green onion, diced
- 1/2 tsp Italian seasoning

Sandwich:

- 1/2 lb bacon, pre-cooked
- 1 small lettuce
- 1 medium tomato sliced
- 1 tbsp mayo

Directions:

1. Preheat your mini waffle maker
2. Whip the egg in a small mixing bowl
3. Add the seasonings, cheese, and onion. Mix thoroughly until it's well incorporated
4. Add a teaspoon of shredded cheese to the waffle maker and cook for 30 seconds

5. Place half the batter in the waffle pan and cook for 4 minutes

6. Once the first chaffle is done, repeat the process with the chaffle

7. Once ready remove and place on a plate. Top with the mayo, lettuce, bacon, and tomato.

8. Place the second chaffle on top, slice into 2 and enjoy!

Nutritional Values: Calories per Servings: 240Kcal: Fats: 18 g : Carbs: 2 g : Protein: 17 g

3. Cauliflower & Italian Seasoning

Servings: 4

Cooking Time: 20 Minutes

Ingredients:

- 1 cup cauliflower rice
- 1/4 teaspoon garlic powder
- 1/2 teaspoon Italian seasoning
- Salt and freshy ground black pepper to taste
- 1/2 cup Parmesan cheese, shredded

Directions:

1. Preheat a mini waffle iron and details, you fit money
2. In a blender, add the Ingredients: except parmesan cheese and pulse until well combined
3. Place 11/2 tablespoon of the Parmesan
4. cheese in the bottom of preheated waffle iron.
5. Place 1/4 of the egg mixture over cheese and sprinkle with the 1/2 tablespoon of the Parmesan cheese.
6. cook for about 4-minutes or until golden brown.
7. Repeat with the remaining mixture and Parmesan cheese.

8. Serve warm.

Nutritional Values: Per Servings: Calories: 12 7Net Carb: 2gFat: 9gSaturated Fat: 5.3gCarbohydrates: 2.7gDietary Fiber: 0.7g Sugar: 1.5gProtein: 9.2g

4. Chaffle Cuban Sandwich

Servings: 1

Cooking Time: 10 minutes

Ingredients:

- 1 Large egg
- 1 Tbsp almond flour
- 1 Tbsp Full-fat greek yogurt
- 1/4 tsp baking powder
- 1/4 cup shredded swiss cheese

For the filling:

- 3 oz roast pork
- 2 oz deli ham
- 1 slice swiss chance
- 3-5 sliced pickle hip
- 3 oz roast pork
- 2 oz deli ham
- 1 slice Swiss cheese
- 3-5 sliced pickle chips
- 1/2 Tbsp Dijon mustard

Directions:

1. Turn on waffle maker to heat and oil it with cooking spray.

2. Beat egg, yogurt, almond flour, and baking powder in a bowl.
3. Sprinkle 1/4 swiss cheese on hot waffle maker. Top with half of the egg mixture, then add 4 of the cheese on top. Close and cook for 5 minutes, until brown and crispy.
4. Repeat with remaining batter.
5. 5. Layer pork, ham, and cheese slice in a small microwaveable bowl. Microwave for seconds, until cheese melts.
6. 6. Spread the inside of chaffle with mustard and top with pickles. Invert bowl onto Chaffle top so that cheese is touching pickles. Place bottom chaffle onto pork and serve.

Nutritional Values: Carbs: 4 g ;Fat: 46 g ;Protein: 33g ;Calories: 522

5. Protein Chaffles

Servings: 1

Cooking Time: 4 Minutes

Ingredients:

- 1/4 cup almond milk
- 1/4 cup plant-based protein powder
- 2 tbsp almond butter
- 1 tbsp psyllium husk

Directions:

1. Preheat the waffle maker.
2. Combine almond milk, protein powder, psyllium husk and mix thoroughly until the mixture gets the form of a paste.
3. Add in butter, combine well and form round balls
4. Place the ball in the center of preheated waffle maker.
5. Cook for 4 minutes.
6. Remove, top as prefer and enjoy.

Nutritional Values: Calories per Servings: 310 Kcai: Fats: 19 g : Carbs: 5 g : Protein: 25 g

6. Garlic powder & Oregano Chaffles

Servings: 2

Cooking Time: 10 Minutes

Ingredients:

- 1/2 cup Mozzarella cheese, grated
- 1 medium organic egg, beaten
- 2 tablespoons almond flour
- 1/2 teaspoon dried oregano, crushed
- 1/2 teaspoon garlic powder
- Salt, to taste

Directions:

1. Preheat a mini waffle iron and then grease it.
2. In a medium bowl, place all Ingredients: and mix until well combined.
3. Place half of the mixture into preheated waffle iron and cook for about 4-5 minutes or until golden brown.
4. Repeat with the remaining mixture.
5. Serve warm.

Nutritional Values: Per Servings: Calories: 100Net Carb: 1.4gFat: 7.2 g Saturated Fat: 1.7gCarbohydrates: 2.4gOietary Fiber: 1g Sugar: O.Protein:4.9g

7. Tuna Chaffles

Servings: 2

Cooking Time: 9 Minutes

Ingredients:

- 1 organic egg, beaten
- 1/2 cup plus 2 teaspoons Mozzarella cheese, shredded and divided
- 1 (2.6-ounce) can water-packed tuna, drained
- Pinch of salt

Directions:

1. Preheat a mini waffle iron and then grease it.
2. In a bowl, place the egg, 1/2 cup of mozzarella cheese, tuna and salt and mix well
3. Place 1 teaspoon of Mozzarella cheese in the bottom of preheated waffle iron and cook for about seconds.
4. Place the egg mixture over cheese and cook for about minutes or until golden brown.
5. Repeat with the remaining mixture.
6. Serve warm.

Nutritional Values: Per Servings: Calories: 94Net Carb: 0.4gFat: 3.Saturated Fat: 1.5 Carbohydrates: 0.4g Dietary Fiber: Og Sugar: 0.2gProtein: 14.2g

8. Sausage & Veggie Chaffles

Servings: 4

Cooking Time: 20 Minutes

Ingredients:

- 1/3 cup unsweetened almond milk.
- 4 medium organic eggs
- 2 tablespoons gluten-free breakfast.
- sausage, cut into slices
- 2 tablespoons broccoli florets, chopped
- 2 tablespoons bell peppers, seeded and chopped
- 2 tablespoons mozzarella cheese, shredded

Directions:

1. Preheat a waffle iron and then grease it.
2. In a medium bowl, add the almond milk 1Z
3. and eggs and beat well.
4. Place the remaining Ingredients: and stir to combine well.
5. Place desired amount of the mixture into
6. preheated waffle iron.
7. Cook for about minutes.
8. Repeat with the remaining
9. Serve warm.

Nutritional Values: Calories 132 Net Carbs 1.2 g Total Fat 9.2 g Saturated Fat 3.5 g Cholesterol 1"]1 117 mg Sodium 216 mg Total Carbs 1.4 g Fiber 0.2 g Sugar 0.5 g Protein 11.1 g

9. Zucchini Chaffles On Pan

Servings: 4

Cooking Time:5minutes

Ingredients:

- 1 cup zucchini, grated
- 1 egg
- 1 cup cheddar cheese
- pinch of salt
- 1 tbsp. avocado oil

Directions:

1. Heat your nonstick pan over medium heat.

2. Pour salt over grated zucchini and let it sit for 5 minutes.

3. Remove water from zucchini

4. In a small bowl, mix zucchini, egg, and cheese together.

5. Grease pan with avocado oil.

6. Once the pan is hot, pour 2 tbsps. zucchini batter and cook for about 12 minutes.

7. Flip and cook for another 1-2 minutes.

8. Once the chaffle is brown, remove from pan.

9. Serve coconut cream on top and enjoy.

Nutritional Values: Per Servings: Protein: 21% 42 kcal
Fat: 77% 153 kcal Carbohydrates: 2% 3 kcal

10.   Bit Chaffle Sandwich

Servings: 1

Cooking Time: 10 Minutes

Ingredients:

Sandwich Filling:

- 2 strips of bacon
- A pinch of salt
- 2 slices tomato
- 1 tbsp mayonnaise
- 3 pieces lettuce

Chaffle:

- 1 egg (beaten)
- 1/2 cup shredded mozzarella cheese
- 1/4 tsp onion powder
- 1/4 tsp garlic powder
- 1/2 tsp curry powder

Directions:

1. Plug the waffle maker and preheat it. Spray it with a non-stick spray.

2. In a mixing bowl, combine the cheese, onion powder, garlic and curry powder. Add the egg and mix until the Ingredients: are well combined.

3. Fill the waffle maker with the batter and spread the batter to the edges of the waffle maker to cover all the holes on the waffle iron.

4. Close the lid of the waffle maker and cook for about minutes or according to waffle maker's settings.

5. After the cooking cycle, remove the chaffle from the waffle maker using a silicone or plastic utensil.

6. Repeat step 3 to 5 until you have cooked all the batter into chaffles. Set the chaffles aside to cool.

7. Heat up a skillet over medium heat. Add the bacon strips and sear until all sides of the bacon is browned, turning and pressing the bacon while searing.

8. Use a slotted spoon to transfer the bacon to a paper towel lined plate to drain.

9. Place the chaffles on a flat surface and spread mayonnaise over the face of the chaffles.

10. Divide the lettuce into two and layer it on one portion on both chaffles.

11. Layer the tomatoes on one of the chaffles and sprinkle with salt. Layer the bacon over the tomatoes and place the other chaffle over the one containing the bacon.

12. Press and serve immediately.

Enjoy!!!

Nutritional Values: Per Servings: Fat 3QB 39% Carbohydrate 7.8g 3% Sugars 2.7g Protein 18.4g

11.   Keto Pepperoni Pizza Chaffle

Servings: 2

Prep time: 10 minutes

Ingredients

- 1 egg
- 1/2 cup mozzarella cheese shredded
- Just a pinch of Italian seasoning
- No sugar added pizza sauce about 1 tablespoon
- Top with more shredded cheese pepperoni

INSTRUCTIONS

1. Preheat the Dash waffle maker.
2. In a small bowl, whip the egg and seasonings together.
3. Mix in the shredded cheese.
4. Add a tsp of shredded cheese to the preheated waffle maker and let it cook for about 30 seconds. This will help to create a more crisp crust.
5. Add half the mixture to the waffle maker and cook it for about 4 minutes until it's golden brown and slightly crispy!
6. Remove the waffle and add the remaining mixture to the waffle maker to make the second chaffle.

2. Top with a tablespoon of pizza sauce, shredded cheese, and pepperoni. Microwave it on high for about 20 seconds and voila! Instant Chaffle PIZZA!

Nutritional Values: Calories: 76kcal Carbohydrates: 4.1g Protein: 5.5g Fat: 4.3g Fiber: 1.2g Sugar: 1.9g

12. Easy Chaffle with Keto Sausage Gravy

Prep time: 5 minutes+ Cook time: 10 minutes

Ingredients

For the Chaffle:

- 1 egg
- 1/2 cup mozzarella cheese, grated
- 1 tsp coconut flour
- 1 tsp water
- 1/4 tsp baking powder
- pinch of salt

For the Keto Sausage Gravy:

- 1/4 cup breakfast sausage, browned
- 3 tbsp chicken broth
- 2 tbsp heavy whipping cream
- 2 tsp cream cheese, softened
- dash garlic powder
- pepper to taste
- dash of onion powder (optional)

Instructions

1. Plug Dash Mini Waffle Maker into the wall and allow to heat up. Grease lightly or use cooking spray.

2. Combine all the ingredients for the chaffle into a small bowl and stir to combine well.
3. Pour half of the chaffle batter onto the waffle maker, then shut the lid and cook for approx 4 minutes.
4. Remove chaffle from waffle maker and repeat the same process to make the second chaffle. Set aside to crisp.

For the Keto Sausage Gravy

5. Cook one pound of breakfast sausage and drain. Reserve 1/4 cup for this .
6. Make sausage patties out of the rest of the sausage and reserve 1/4 a cup to brown for this . If you aren't familiar with breakfast sausage, it is crumbled like ground beef.
2. Wipe excess grease from the skillet and add 1/4 cup browned breakfast sausage and the rest of the ingredients and bring to a boil stirring continuously.
3. Reduce heat to medium and continue to cook down with the lid off so that it begins to thicken for approximately 5-7 minutes. If you'd like it very thick, you can add a bit of Xanthan Gum, but if you are patient with it simmering the keto sausage gravy will thicken. Then, it will thicken even more as it cools.

4. Add salt and pepper to taste and spoon keto sausage gravy over chaffles.

5. Enjoy

Nutritional Values: Calories: 212kcal Carbohydrates: 3g Protein: 11g Fat: 17g Saturated Fat: 10g Cholesterol: 134mg Sodium: 350mg Potassium: 133mg Fiber: 1g Sugar: 1g Vitamin A: 595IU Vitamin C: 2mg Calcium: 191mg Iron: 1mg

13. BLT Keto Chaffle Sandwich

Servings: 1

Prep time: 3 minutes + Cook time: 10 minutes

INGREDIENTS

For the chaffles

- 1 egg
- 1/2 cup Cheddar cheese, shredded

For the sandwich

- 2 strips bacon
- 1-2 slices tomato
- 2-3 pieces lettuce
- 1 tablespoon mayonnaise

INSTRUCTIONS

1. Preheat the waffle maker according to manufacturer instructions.
2. In a small mixing bowl, mix together egg and shredded cheese. Stir until well combined.
3. Pour one half of the waffle batter into the waffle maker. Cook for 3-4 minutes or until golden brown. Repeat with the second half of the batter.

2. In a large pan over medium heat, cook the bacon until crispy, turning as needed. Remove to drain on paper towels.
3. Assemble the sandwich with lettuce, tomato, and mayonnaise. Enjoy!

NOTES

If you are using a larger size waffle maker, you may be able to cook the whole amount of batter in one waffle. This will vary with the size of your machine.

Nutritional Values: CALORIES: 238 TOTAL FAT: 18g SATURATED FAT: 9g TRANS FAT: 0g UNSATURATED FAT: 7g CHOLESTEROL: 143mg SODIUM: 554mg CARBOHYDRATES: 2g FIBER: 0g SUGAR: 1g PROTEIN: 17g

14.   Mini Keto Pizza

Servings: 2

Prep time: 5 minutes+ Cook time: 10 minutes

Ingredients

- 1/2 cup Shredded Mozzarella cheese
- 1 tablespoon almond flour
- 1/2 tsp baking powder
- 1 egg
- 1/4 tsp garlic powder
- 1/4 tsp basil
- 2 tablespoons low carb pasta sauce
- 2 tablespoons mozzarella cheese

Instructions

1. While the waffle maker is heating up, in a bowl mix mozzarella cheese, baking powder, garlic, basis, egg and almond flour.
2. 1/2 the mixture into your mini waffle maker.
3. Cook for 3-5 minutes until your pizza waffle is completely cooked. If you check it and the waffle sticks to the waffle maker let it cook for another minute or two.

4. Next put the remainder of the pizza crust mix into the waffle maker and cook it.
5. Once both pizza crusts are cooked, place them on the baking sheet of your toaster oven.
6. Put 1 tablespoon of low carb pasta sauce on top of each pizza crust.
7. Sprinkle 1 tablespoon of shredded mozzarella cheese on top of each one.
8. Bake at 350 degrees in the toaster oven for roughly 5 minutes, just until the cheese is melted.

Nutritional Values: Calories: 195kcal | Carbohydrates: 4g | Protein: 13g | Fat: 14g | Saturated Fat: 6g | Cholesterol: 116mg | Sodium: 301mg | Potassium: 178mg | Fiber: 1g | Sugar: 1g | Vitamin A: 408IU | Calcium: 290mg | Iron: 1mg

15. Keto Chaffle Italian Garlic And Herb

Servings: 1

Prep Time: 5 minutes+ Cook Time: 3-5 minutes

Ingredients

- ½ C. Shredded mozzarella cheese
- 1 Egg
- 1 Tbsp. Almond flour
- ¼ tsp. Garlic powder
- ¼ tsp. Italian seasoning
- 1 Tbsp. Heavy whipping cream
- ¼ C. Grated parmesan cheese
- Mini waffle maker

Instructions

1. Preheat your mini waffle maker.
2. Mix together the ingredients for the chaffle in a mixing bowl until completely combined. This mixture will not be liquid like most waffle batters, it is supposed to have a more solid consistency.
3. Spread half of the mixture evenly into the mini waffle maker, and cook for 3-5 minutes until it is done to your liking.

4. Remove the first chaffle, and put the second half of the batter into the mini waffle maker.
5. Eat your chaffles as they are, or make them into a sandwich with your favorite keto-friendly options. We used a baked Italian herb chicken with fresh veggies for a healthy meal.

Nutritional Values: Net Carbs: 6 net carbs per serving

16.   Easy Sandwich Chaffle

Servings: 2

Prep time: 10 minutes

Ingredients

- 2 egg whites
- 2 teaspoons of water
- 2 tbsp cream cheese I had light cream cheese
- 4 tbsp ground almonds
- 1/4 tsp baking powder
- 1 pinch of salt

Instructions

1. Mix all ingredients together and bake in portions in the waffle iron. I got four mini chaffles from the .

Nutritional Values: Calories: 72 kcal Carbohydrates: 1 g Protein: 4 g Fat: 5 g

17. Aioli Chicken Chaffle Sandwich

Servings: 1

Cooking Time: 6 Minutes

Ingredients:

- l/4 cup shredded rotisserie chicken
- 2 Tbsp Kewpie mayo
- 1/2 tsp lemon juice
- 1 grated garlic clove
- 1/4 green onion, chopped
- 1egg
- 1/2 cup shredded mozzarella cheese

Directions:

1. Mix lemon juice and mayo in a small bowl.
2. Turn on waffle maker to heat and oil it with cooking spray.
3. Beat eggs in a small bowl.
4. Place 1/8 cup of cheese on waffle maker, then spread half of the egg mixture over it and top with 1/8 cup of cheese. Close and cook for 3-minutes.
5. Repeat for remaining batter.
6. Place chicken on chaffles and top with sauce. Sprinkle with chopped green onion.

Nutritional Values: Carbs: 3 g ;Fat: 42 g ;Protein: 34 g
;Calories: 545

18. Sage & Coconut Milk Chaffles

Servings: 6

Cooking Time: 24 Minutes

Ingredients:

- 3/4 cup coconut flour, sifted
- 1 1/2 teaspoons organic baking powder
- 1/2 teaspoon dried ground sage
- 1/8 teaspoon garlic powder
- 1/8 teaspoon salt
- 1 organic egg
- 1 cup unsweetened coconut milk
- 1/4cup water
- 1/2 tablespoons coconut oil, melted
- 1/2 cup cheddar cheese, shredded

Directions:

1. Preheat a waffle iron and then grease it.
2. In a bowl, add the flour, baking powder, sage, garlic powder and salt and mix well.
3. Add the egg, coconut milk, water and coconut oil and mix until a stiff mixture forms.
4. Add the cheese and gently stir to combine.

5. Divide the mixture into 6 portions.
6. Place 1 portion of the mixture into preheated waffle iron and cook for about 4 minutes or until golden brown.
7. Repeat with the remaining
8. Serve warm.

Nutritional Values: Per Servings: Calories: 147Net . Carb: 2.2gFat: 13 gSaturated Fat: 10.7gCarbohydrates: 2.Dietary Fiber: 0.7g Sugar: 1.3gProtein: 4g

19.   Chaffle Burger

Servings: 1

Cooking Time: 10 Minutes

Ingredients:

For the burger:

- 1/3-pound ground beef
- 1/2 tsp garlic salt
- 2 slices American cheese

For the chaffles:

- 1 large egg
- 1/2 cup shredded mozzarella
- 1/4 tsp garlic salt

For the sauce:

- 2 tsp mayonnaise
- 1 tsp ketchup
- 1 tsp dill pickle relish
- splash vinegar, to taste

For the TOPPINGs:

- 2 Tbsp shredded lettuce
- 3-4 dill pickles

- 2 tsp onion, minced

Directions:

1. Heat a griddle over medium-high heat.
2. Divide ground beef into balls and place on the griddle, 6 inches apart. cook for 1 minute.
3. Use a small plate to flatten beef. Sprinkle with garlic salt.
4. cook for 2-3, until halfway cooked through. Flip and sprinkle with garlic salt.
5. cook for 2-3 minutes, or until cooked completely.
6. Place cheese slice over each patty and stack patties. Set aside on a plate. Cover with foil.
7. Turn on waffle maker to heat and oil it with cooking spray.
8. whisk egg, cheese, and garlic salt until well combined.
9. Add half of the egg mixture to waffle maker and cook for 2-3 minutes.
10. Set aside and repeat with remaining batter.
11. whisk all sauce Ingredients: in a bowl.

12. Top one chaffle with the stacked burger patties, shredded lettuce, pickles, and onions.

13. Spread sauce over the other chaffle and place sauce side down over the sandwich.

14. Eat immediately.

Nutritional Values: Carbs: 8 g ;Fat: 5 6 g ;Protein: 6 5 g ;Calories: 831

20.   Hot Ham Chaffle

Servings: 2

Cooking Time: 4 Minutes

Ingredients:

- 1/2 cup mozzarella cheese, shredded
- 1 egg
- 1/4 cup ham, chopped
- 1/4 tsp salt
- 2 tbsp mayonnaise
- 1 tsp Dijon mustard

Directions:

1. Preheat your waffle iron.
2. In the meantime, add the egg in a small mixing bowl and whisk.
3. Add in the ham, cheese, combine.
4. Scoop half the mixture using a spoon and pour into the hot waffle iron.
5. Close and cook for 4 minutes.
6. Remove the waffle and place on a large plate. Repeat the process with the remaining batter.
7. In a separate small bowl, add the mayo and mustard. Mix together until smooth.

8. Slice the waffles in quarters and use the mayo mixture as the dip.

Nutritional Values: Calories per Servings: 110 Kcal; Fats: 12 g ; Carbs: 6 g ; Protein: 12 g

21. Vegan Chaffle

Servings: 1

Cooking Time: 25 Minutes

Ingredients:

- 1 Tbsp flaxseed meal
- 2 1/2 Tbsp water
- 1/4 cup low carb vegan cheese
- 2 Tbsp coconut flour
- 1 Tbsp low carb vegan cream cheese, softened
- Pinch of salt

Directions:

1. Turn on waffle maker to heat and oil it, with cooking spray.
2. Mix flaxseed and water in a bowl. Leave for 5 minutes, until thickened and gooey.
3. whisk remaining Ingredients: for Chaffle.
4. Pour one half of the batter into the center of the waffle maker. Close and cook for 3 - 5 minutes.
5. Remove chaffle and serve.

Nutritional Values: Carbs: 3 3 g ;Fat: 2 5 g ;protein: 25 g ;Calories:450

22.   Broccoli And Cheese

Servings: 1

Cooking Time: 5 Minutes

Ingredients:

- 1/3 cup raw broccoli, finely chopped
- 1/4 cup shredded cheddar cheese
- 1 egg
- 1/2 tsp garlic powder
- 1/2 tsp dried minced onion
- Salt and pepper, to taste

Directions:

1. Turn on waffle maker to heat the oil it with cooking spray
2. Beat egg in a small bowl
3. Fold in cheese, broccoli, onion, garlic powder, salt and pepper
4. Pour egg mixture into waffle maker. Cook for minutes, or until done.
5. Remove from waffle maker with a fork
6. Serve with sour cream and butter.

Nutritional Values: Carbs: 4 g ;Fat: 9 g ;Protein: g ;Calories: 125

23. Lemon Fresh Herbs Chaffles

Servings: 6

Cooking Time: 24 Minutes

Ingredients:

- 1/2 cup ground flaxseed
- 2 organic eggs
- 1/2 cup goat cheddar cheese, grated
- 2-4 tablespoons plain Greek yogurt
- 1 tablespoon avocado oil
- 1/2 teaspoon baking soda
- 1 teaspoon fresh lemon juice
- 2 tablespoons fresh chives, minced
- 1 tablespoon fresh basil, minced
- 1/2 tablespoon fresh mint, minced
- 1/4 tablespoon fresh thyme, minced
- 1/4 tablespoon fresh oregano, minced
- Salt and freshly ground black pepper, to taste

Directions:

1. Preheat a waffle iron and then grease it.
2. In a medium bowl, place all Ingredients: and with a fork, mix until well combined.
3. Divide the mixture into 6 portions.

4. Place 1 portion of the mixture into preheated waffle iron and cook for about minutes or until golden brown.
5. Repeat with the remaining
6. Serve warm.

Nutritional Values1Per Servings: Calories: 11et · Carb: 0.9gFat: 7.9gSaturated Fat: 3g Carbohydrates: 3.7gDietary Fiber: 2.8g Sugar: 0.7gPro- g protein: 6.4g

24. Italian Seasoning Chaffles

Servings: 2

Cooking Time: 8 Minutes

Ingredients:

- 1/2 cup Mozzarella cheese, shredded
- 1 tablespoon Parmesan cheese, shredded
- 1 organic egg
- 3/4 teaspoon coconut flour
- 1/4 teaspoon organic baking powder
- 1/8 teaspoon Italian seasoning
- Pinch of salt

Directions:

1. Preheat a mini waffle iron and then grease It.
2. In a medium bowl, place all Ingredients: and with a fork, mix until well combined.
3. Place half of the mixture into preheated waffle iron and cook for about 4 minutes or until golden brown.
4. Repeat with the remaining mixture.
5. Serve warm.

Nutritional Values: Per Servings: Calories: Bet Carb: 1.9 gFat: 5 g Saturated Fat: 2.6 g Carbohydrates: 3.8 g Dietary Fiber: 1.9 g Sugar: 0.6gProtein: 6.5g

25. Basil Chaffles

Servings: 3

Cooking Time: 16 Minutes

Ingredients:

- 2 organic eggs, beaten
- 1/2 cup Mozzarella cheese, shredded
- 1 tablespoon Parmesan cheese, grated
- 1 teaspoon dried basil, crushed
- Pinch of salt

Directions:

1. Preheat a mini waffle iron and then grease it.
2. In a medium bowl, place all Ingredients: and mix until well combined.
3. Place l/of the mixture into preheated waffle iron and cook for about 3-4 minutes or until golden brown.
4. Repeat with the remaining mixture
5. Serve warm.

Nutritional Values: Per Servings: Calories: Net Cull: OAg Fat: 4.2gSaturated Fat: 1.6gCarbohydrates:

0.4g Dietary Fiber: Og Sugar: 0.2gProtein: 5.7g

26. Lt Chaffle Sandwich

Servings: 2

Cooking Time: 15 Minutes

Ingredients:

- Cooking spray
- 4 slices bacon
- 1 tablespoon mayonnaise
- 4 basic chaffles
- 2 lettuce leaves
- 2 tomato slices

Directions:

1. Coat your pan with foil and place it over medium heat.

2. Cook the bacon until golden and crispy.

3. Spread mayo on top of the chaffle.

4. Top with the lettuce, bacon and tomato.

5. Top with another chaffle.

Nutritional Values: Calories 238 Total Fat 18.4g Saturated Fat 5. Cholesterol 44mg Sodium 931mg Potassium

258mg Total Carbohydrate 39 Dietary Fiber o.2g Protein 14.3g Total Sugars 0.99

27. Mozzarella Peanut Butter Chaffle

Servings: 2

Cooking Time: 15 Minutes

Ingredients:

- 1 egg, lightly beaten
- 2 tbsp peanut butter
- 2 tbsp Swerve
- 1/2 cup mozzarella cheese, shredded

Directions:

1. Preheat your waffle maker.

2. In a bowl, mix egg, cheese, Swerve, and peanut butter until well combined.

3. Spray waffle maker with cooking spray.

4. Pour half batter in the hot waffle maker and cook for minutes or until golden brown. Repeat with the remaining batter.

5. Serve and enjoy.

Nutritional Values: Calories 15oFat 11.5 g Carbohydrates 5.g Sugar 1.7 gProtein8.8 g Cholesterol 86 mg

28. Sausage & Pepperoni Chaffle Sandwich

Servings: 4

Cooking Time: 10 Minutes

Ingredients:

- Cooking spray
- 2 cervelat sausage, sliced into rounds
- 12 pieces pepperoni
- 6 mushroom slices
- 4 teaspoons mayonnaise
- 4 big white onion rings
- 4 basic chaffles

Directions:

1. Spray your skillet with oil.

2. Place over medium heat.

3. Cook the sausage until brown on both sides.

4. Transfer on a plate.

5. Cook the pepperoni and mushrooms for 2 minutes.

6. Spread mayo on top of the chaffle.

7. Top with the sausage, pepperoni, mushrooms and onion rings.

8. Top with another chaffle.

Nutritional Values: Calories 373 Total Fat 24.4g Saturated Fat 6g Cholesterol 27Ing Sodium 717Ing Potassium 105mg Total Carbohydrate 28g Dietary Fiber 1.1g Protein 8.g Total Sugars 4.59

29.   Pizza Flavored Chaffle

Servings: 3

Cooking Time: 12 Minutes

Ingredients:

- 1 egg, beaten
- 1/2 cup cheddar cheese, shredded
- 2 tablespoons pepperoni, chopped
- 1 tablespoon keto marinara sauce
- 4 tablespoons almond flour
- 1 teaspoon baking powder
- 1/2 teaspoon dried Italian seasoning
- Parmesan cheese, grated

Directions:

1. Preheat your waffle maker.

2. In a bowl, mix the egg, cheddar cheese, pepperoni, marinara sauce, almond flour, baking powder and Italian seasoning.

3. Add the mixture to the waffle maker.

4. Close the device and cook for minutes.

5. Open it and transfer chaffle to a plate.

6. Let cool for 2 minutes.

7. Repeat the steps with the remaining batter.

8. Top with the grated Parmesan and serve.

Nutritional Values: Calories 17 Total Fat14.3g Saturated Fat 7.59 Cholesterol 118mg Sodium 3oomg Potassium 326mg Total Carbohydrate 1.8g Dietary Fiber o.lg Protein 11.1g Total Sugars 0.49

30.   Italian Sausage Chaffles

Servings: 2

Cooking Time: 8 Minutes

Ingredients:

- 1 egg, beaten
- 1 cup cheddar cheese, shredded
- 1/4 cup Parmesan cheese, grated
- 1 lb. Italian sausage, crumbled
- 2 teaspoons baking powder
- 1 cup almond flour

Directions:

1. Preheat your waffle maker.

2. Mix all the Ingredients: in a bowl.

3. Pour half of the mixture into the waffle maker.

4. Cover and cook for minutes.

5. Transfer to a plate.

6. Let cool to make it crispy.

7. Do the same steps to make the next chaffle.

Nutritional Values: Calories 332 Total Fat

27.1g Saturated Fat 10.2g Cholesterol 99 Sodium 634mg
Total Carbohydrate 1.99 Dietary Fiber o.5g Total Sugars
o.lg Protein ig.6g Potassium 359mg

31. Bacon, Olives & Cheddar Chaffle

Servings: 2

Cooking Time: 8 Minutes

Ingredients:

- 1 egg
- 1/2 cup cheddar cheese, shredded
- 1 tablespoon black olives, chopped
- 1 tablespoon bacon bits

Directions:

1. Plug in your waffle maker.

2. In a bowl, beat the egg and stir in the cheese.

3. Add the black olives and bacon bits.

4. Mix well.

5. Add half of the mixture into the waffle maker.

6. Cover and cook for 4 minutes.

7. Open and transfer to a plate.

8. Let cool for 2 minutes.

9. Cook the other chaffle using the remaining batter.

Nutritional Values: Calories 202 Total Fat i6g Saturated Fat 8g Cholesterol 122mg Sodium 462mg Potassium 111mg Total Carbohydrate o.gg Dietary Fiber 0.1g Protein 13.4g Total Sugars 0.39

32. Zucchini Chaffle

Servings: 2

Cooking Time: 8 Minutes

Ingredients:

- 1 cup zucchini, grated
- 1/4 cup mozzarella cheese, shredded
- 1 egg, beaten
- 1/2 cup Parmesan cheese, shredded
- 1 teaspoon dried basil
- Salt and pepper to taste

Directions:

1. Preheat your waffle maker.

2. Sprinkle pinch of salt over the zucchini and mix.

3. Let sit for 2 minutes.

4. Wrap zucchini with paper towel and squeeze to get rid of water.

5. Transfer to a bowl and stir in the rest of the Ingredients.

6. Pour half of the mixture into the waffle maker.

7. Close the device.

8. Cook for 4 minutes.

9. Make the second chaffle following the same steps.

Nutritional Values: Calories 194 Total Fat 13 g Saturated Fat 7 g Cholesterol 115 mg Sodium 789 mg Potassium 223 mg Total Carbohydrate 4 g Dietary Fiber 1 g Protein 16 g Total Sugars 2 g

33.   Chicken Quesadilla Chaffle

Servings: 2

Cooking Time: 14 Minutes

Ingredients:

- 1 egg, beaten
- 1/4 tsp taco seasoning
- 1/3 cup finely grated cheddar cheese
- 1/3 cup cooked chopped chicken

Directions:

1. Preheat the waffle iron.

2. In a medium bowl, mix the eggs, taco seasoning, and cheddar cheese. Add the chicken and combine well.

3. Open the iron, lightly grease with cooking spray and pour in half of the mixture.

4. Close the iron and cook until brown and crispy, 7 minutes.

5. Remove the chaffle onto a plate and set aside.

6. Make another chaffle using the remaining mixture.

7. Serve afterward.

Nutritional Values: Per Servings: Calories 314 Fats 20.64g Carbs 5.719Net Carbs 5.71g Protein 16.74g

34. Chicken Chaffle Sandwich

Servings: 2

Cooking Time: 15 Minutes

Ingredients:

- 1 chicken breast fillet, sliced into strips
- Salt and pepper to taste
- 1 teaspoon dried rosemary
- 1 tablespoon olive oil
- 4 basic chaffles
- 2 tablespoons butter, melted
- 2 tablespoons Parmesan cheese, grated

Directions:

1. Season the chicken strips with salt, pepper and rosemary.

2. Add olive oil to a pan over medium low heat.

3. Cook the chicken until brown on both sides.

4. Spread butter on top of each chaffle.

5. Sprinkle cheese on top.

6. Place the chicken on top and top with another chaffle.

Nutritional Values: Calories 262 Total Fat 2og Saturated Fat 9.2g Cholesterol mg Sodium 27omg Potassium 125mg Total Carbohydrate 1g Dietary Fiber o.2g Protein 20.2g Total Sugars 0g

35. Cheese Garlic Chaffle

Servings: 2

Cooking Time: 8 Minutes

Ingredients:

Chaffle:

- 1 egg
- 1 teaspoon cream cheese
- 1/2 cup mozzarella cheese, shredded
- 1/2 teaspoon garlic powder
- 1 teaspoon Italian seasoning

TOPPING:

- 1 tablespoon butter
- 1/2 teaspoon garlic powder
- 1/2 teaspoon Italian seasoning
- 2 tablespoon mozzarella cheese, shredded

Directions:

1. Plug in your waffle maker to preheat.

2. Preheat your oven to 350 degrees F.

3. In a bowl, combine all the chaffle Ingredients.

4. Cook in the waffle maker for minutes per chaffle.

5. Transfer to a baking pan.

6. Spread butter on top of each chaffle.

7. Sprinkle garlic powder and Italian seasoning on top.

8. Top with mozzarella cheese.

9. Bake until the cheese has melted.

Nutritional Values: Calories141 Total Fat 13 g Saturated Fat 8 g Cholesterol 115.8 mg Sodium 255.8 mg Potassium 350 mg Total Carbohydrate 2.6g Dietary Fiber 0.79

36.   Best Keto Pizza Chaffle

Servings: 2

Prep Time: 5 mins

Cook Time: 15 mins

Ingredients:

- 1 tsp coconut flour
- 1 egg white
- 1/2 cup mozzarella cheese, shredded
- 1 tsp cream cheese, softened
- 1/4 tsp baking powder
- 1/8 tsp Italian seasoning
- 1/8 tsp garlic powder
- pinch of salt
- 3 tsp low carb marinara sauce
- 1/2 cup mozzarella cheese
- 6 pepperonis cut in half
- 1 tbsp parmesan cheese, shredded
- 1/4 tsp basil seasoning

Directions:

1. Preheat oven to 400 degrees. Turn waffle maker on or plug it in so that it gets hot.

2. In a small bowl add coconut flour, egg white, mozzarella cheese, softened cream cheese, baking powder, garlic powder, Italian seasonings, and a pinch of salt.
3. Pour 1/2 of the batter in the waffle maker, close the top, and cook for 3-4 minutes or until chaffle reaches desired doneness.
4. Carefully remove chaffle from the waffle maker, then follow the same Directions: to make the second chaffle.
5. Top each chaffle with tomato sauce (I used 1 1/2 tsp per), pepperoni, mozzarella cheese, and parmesan cheese.
6. Place in the oven on a baking sheet (or straight on the baking rack) on the top shelf of the oven for 5-6 minutes. Then turn the oven to broil so that the cheese begins to bubble and brown. Keep a close eye as it can burn quickly. I broiled my pizza chaffle for approx 1 min and 30 seconds.
7. Remove from oven and sprinkle basil on top.
8. Enjoy!

Nutritional values: Calories: 241kcal | Carbohydrates: 4g | Protein: 17g | Fat: 18g | Saturated Fat: 10g | Cholesterol: 49mg | Sodium: 430mg | Potassium:

130mg | Fiber: 1g | Sugar: 1g | Vitamin A: 412IU | Calcium: 339mg | Iron: 1mg

37.   Keto Taco Chaffle with Crispy Taco Shells

Servings: 1

Prep Time: 5 minutes+ Cook Time: 8 mins

Ingredients:

- 1 egg white
- 1/4 cup Monterey jack cheese, shredded (packed tightly)
- 1/4 cup sharp cheddar cheese, shredded (packed tightly)
- 3/4 tsp water
- 1 tsp coconut flour
- 1/4 tsp baking powder
- 1/8 tsp chili powder
- pinch of salt

Directions:

1. Plug the Dash Mini Waffle Maker in the wall and grease lightly once it is hot.
2. Combine all of the Ingredients: in a bowl and stir to combine.
3. Spoon out 1/2 of the batter on the waffle maker and close lid. Set a timer for 4 minutes and do not lift the lid until the cooking time is complete. If you

do, it will look like the taco chaffle shell isn't setting up properly, but it will. You have to let it cook the entire 4 minutes before lifting the lid.

4. Remove the taco chaffle shell from the waffle iron and set aside. Repeat the same steps above with the rest of the chaffle batter.

5. Turn over a muffin pan and set the taco chaffle shells between the cups to form a taco shell. Allow to set for a few minutes.

6. Remove and serve with the Very Best Taco Meat or your favorite.

7. Enjoy this delicious keto crispy taco chaffle shell with your favorite TOPPINGs.

Nutritional values: Calories: 258kcal | Carbohydrates: 4g | Protein: 18g | Fat: 19g | Fiber: 2g | Sugar: 1g

38. White Bread Keto Chaffle | Wonder Bread Chaffle

Serving: 2

Prep time: 2 minutes+ cook time: 8 minutes

Ingredients:

- 1 Egg
- 3 tbsp Almond Flour
- 1 tbsp Mayonnaise
- 1/4 tsp Baking Powder
- 1 tsp Water

Directions:

1. Preheat mini waffle maker.
2. In a bowl, whisk the egg until beaten.
3. Add almond flour, mayonnaise, baking powder, and water.
4. When the waffle maker is heated, carefully pour 1/2 of the batter in the waffle maker and close the top. Allow to cook for 3-5 minutes.
5. Carefully remove from the waffle maker and set aside for 2-3 minutes to crisp up.
6. Repeat Directions: do it again for the second chaffle.

Nutrition Values Per Serving: CALORIES: 125 |TOTAL FAT: 11.5g |CARBOHYDRATES: 2g |NET CARBOHYDRATES: 1g| FIBER: 1g |PROTEIN: 5g

39. Keto Rye Bread Chaffle

Serving: 1

Prep Time: 15-20 minutes

INGREDIENTS:

- 1 egg
- 2 tablespoons almond flour
- 1 tablespoon melted butter
- 1 tablespoon mozzarella cheese
- pinch salt
- pinch garlic powder
- 1/2 teaspoon baking powder
- 1/2 teaspoon caraway seeds

DIRECTIONS:

1. Preheat mini waffle maker.
2. Mix all rye bread chaffle Ingredients: in a small bowl.
3. Place 1/2 the mixture into a preheated mini waffle maker.
4. Cook for 4 minutes.
5. Serve warm.

Nutrition Values:Calories: 263kcal |Carbohydrates: 3.1g
|Protein: 10.6g |Fat: 18.8g |Fiber: 0.6g |Sugar: 0.8g
CALORIES: 263 kcal

40. Jalapeno Popper Grilled Cheese Chaffle

Serving: 4

Prep time: 15-20 minutes

INGREDIENTS:

- 2 Jalapenos sliced lengthwise seeds and membranes removed
- 4 ounces cream cheese
- 4 slices bacon crispy cooked
- 2 slices Monterey jack
- 2 slices sharp cheddar

Chaffle Ingredients:

- 2 eggs
- 1 cup mozzarella shredded

DIRECTIONS:

1. Fill each jalapeno half with approximately 1 ounce of cream cheese.
2. Bake stuffed jalapenos in a preheated Air fryer for 10 minutes at 350*.
3. Build your sandwiches: Place 1 slice each Monterey Jack on 2 Chaffles, add 2 jalapeño halves to each, 2 slices of bacon, then cheddar cheese. Top with the other 2 Chaffles.

4. Butter each side of the sandwiches. Grill each side until lightly browned.

TIP: Use gloves to cut the peppers and remove the seeds. Wash hands thoroughly after working with them as they can be an irritant if you touch your face or eyes.

41. Zucchini Nut Bread Chaffle

Serving: 2

Prep time: 20 minutes

INGREDIENTS:

- 1 cup shredded zucchini approximately 1 small zucchini
- 1 egg
- 1/2 teaspoon cinnamon
- 1 Tbsp plus 1 tsp erythritol blend such as Swerve, Pyure or Lakanto
- Dash ground nutmeg
- 2 tsp melted butter
- 1 ounce softened cream cheese
- 2 tsp coconut flour
- 1/2 tsp baking powder
- 3 tablespoons chopped walnuts or pecans
- Frosting Ingredients:
- 2 ounces cream cheese at room temperature
- 2 Tbsp butter at room temperature
- 1/4 tsp cinnamon
- 2 Tbsp caramel sugar-free syrup such as Skinny Girl, OR 1 Tbsp confectioner's sweetener, such as Swerve plus 1/8 tsp caramel extract

- 1 Tbsp chopped walnuts or pecans

DIRECTIONS:

1. Grate zucchini and place in a colander over a plate to drain for 15 minutes. With your hands, squeeze out as much moisture as possible.
2. Preheat mini Dash waffle iron until thoroughly hot.
3. In a medium bowl, whisk all chaffle Ingredients: together until well combined.
4. Spoon a heaping 2 tablespoons of batter into waffle iron, close and cook 3-5 minutes, until done.
5. Remove to a wire rack. Repeat 3 times.
6. Frosting Directions:
7. Mix all Ingredients: together until smooth and spread over each chaffle.
8. Top with additional chopped nuts.

42.   Easy Turkey Burger with Halloumi Cheese Chaffle

Serving: 2

Prep time: 20 minutes

Ingredients:

- 1 lb Ground Turkey raw (no need to precook the turkey)
- 8 oz Halloumi shredded
- 1 zucchini medium, shredded
- 2 tbsp Chives chopped
- 1/2 tsp Salt
- 1/4 tsp Pepper

DIRECTIONS:

1. Add all Ingredients: to a bowl mix thoroughly together.
2. Shape into 8 evenly sized patties
3. Preheat mini griddle.
4. Cook the patties 5-7 minutes

43.   Halloumi Cheese Chaffle

Serving: 3

Prep time: 15 minutes

Ingredients:

- 3 oz Halloumi cheese
- 2 T Pasta sauce optional

DIRECTIONS:

1. Cut Halloumi cheese into 1/2 inch thick slices.
2. Place cheese in the UNHEATED waffle maker.
3. Turn waffle maker on.
4. Let it cook for about 3-6 minutes or until golden
5. brown and to your liking.
6. Let cool on a rack for a few minutes.
7. Add Low Carb marinara or pasta sauce.
8. Serve immediately. Enjoy!

44.   Keto Taco Chaffle

Serving: 3

Prep time: 30 minutes

Ingredients:

- Chaffle Ingredients:
- 1/2 cup cheese cheddar or mozzarella, shredded
- 1 egg
- 1/4 tsp Italian seasoning
- Taco Meat Seasonings Ingredients: for 1 lbs of ground beef
- 1 teaspoon chili powder
- 1 teaspoon ground cumin
- 1/2 teaspoon garlic powder
- 1/2 teaspoon cocoa powder
- 1/4 teaspoon onion powder
- 1/4 teaspoon salt
- 1/12 teaspoon smoked paprika
- Taco Meat Seasoning Ingredients: for Big Batches
- 1/4 cup chili powder
- 1/4 cup ground cumin
- 2 tablespoons garlic powder
- 2 tablespoons cocoa powder
- 1 tablespoon onion powder

- 1 tablespoon salt
- 1 teaspoon smoked paprika

DIRECTIONS:

1. Cook your ground beef or ground turkey first.
2. Add all the taco meat seasonings. The cocoa powder is optional but it totally enhances the flavors of all the other seasonings!
3. While you are making the taco meat, start making the keto chaffles.
4. Preheat the waffle maker. I use a mini waffle maker.
5. In a small bowl, whip the egg first.
6. Add the shredded cheese and seasoning.
7. Place half the chaffle mixture into the mini waffle maker and cook it for about 3 to 4minutes.
8. Repeat and cook the second half of the mixture to make the second chaffle.
9. Add the warm taco meat to your taco chaffle.
10. Top it with lettuce, tomatoes, cheese, and serve warm!

NOTES

I tend to make this in big batches so I always have some on hand! I keep it in mason jars that I can seal and keep in my kitchen pantry. Just add a little label to it and you are good to go. It's so easy to make taco meat seasonings that there's no real reason to purchase the premade taco seasoning packets because they are loaded with not so good Ingredients.

45. Ham Sandwich Chaffles

Servings: 2

Cooking Time: 8 Minutes

Ingredients:

- 1 organic egg, beaten
- 1/2 cup Monterrey Jack cheese, shredded
- 1 teaspoon coconut flour
- Pinch of garlic powder
- Filling
- 2 sugar-free ham slices
- 1 small tomato, sliced
- 2 lettuce leaves

Directions:

1. Preheat a mini waffle iron and then grease it.

2. For chaffles: In a medium bowl, put all Ingredients: and with a fork, mix until well combined. Place half of the mixture into preheated waffle iron and cook for about 3-4 minutes.

3. Repeat with the remaining mixture.

4. Serve each chaffle with filling Ingredients.

Nutritional Values: Calories 1 Net Carbs 3.7 g Total Fat 8.7 g Saturated Fat 3.4 g Cholesterol 114 mg Sodium 794 mg Total Carbs 5.5 g Fiber: 1.8 g Sugar 1.5 g Protein 13.9 g

46.   Chicken Sandwich Chaffles

Servings: 2

Cooking Time: 8 minutes

Ingredients:

- Chaffles
- 1 large organic egg, beaten
- 1/2 cup cheddar cheese, shredded
- Pinch of salt and ground black pepper
- Filling
- 1 (6-ounce) cooked chicken breast, halved
- 2 lettuce leaves
- 1/4 of small onion, sliced
- 1 small tomato, sliced

Directions:

1. Preheat a mini waffle iron and then grease it.
2. For chaffles: In a medium bowl, put all Ingredients: and with a fork, mix until well combined.
3. Place half of the mixture into preheated waffle iron and cook for about 3-4 minutes.
4. Repeat with the remaining mixture.
5. Serve each chaffle with filling Ingredients.

Nutritional Values: Calories 2 Net Carbs 2.5 g Total Fat 14.1 g Saturated Fat 6.8 g Cholesterol 177 mg Sodium 334 mg Total Carbs 3.3 g Fiber 0.8 g Sugar 2 g Protein 28.7 g

47. Salmon & Cheese Sandwich Chaffles

Servings: 4

Cooking Time: 24 minutes

Ingredients:

- Chaffles
- 2 organic eggs
- 1/2 ounce butter, melted
- 1 cup mozzarella cheese, shredded
- 2 tablespoons almond flour
- Pinch of salt
- Filling
- 1/2 cup smoked salmon
- 1/3 cup avocado, peeled, pitted, and sliced
- 2 tablespoons feta cheese, crumbled

Directions:

1. Preheat a mini waffle iron and then grease it.

2. For chaffles: In a medium bowl, put all Ingredients: and with a fork, mix until well combined. Place 1/4 of the mixture into preheated waffle iron and cook for about 5-6 minutes.

3. Repeat with the remaining mixture.

4. Serve each chaffle with filling Ingredients.

Nutritional Values: Calories 16g Net Carbs 1.2 g Total Fat 13.g Saturated Fat 5 g Cholesterol 101 mg Sodium 319 mg Total Carbs 2.8 g Fiber 1.6 g Sugar 0.6 g Protein 8.g

48. Strawberry Cream Cheese Sandwich Chaffles

Servings: 2

Cooking Time: 10 minutes

Ingredients:

Chaffles

- 1 organic egg, beaten
- 1 teaspoon organic vanilla extract
- 1 tablespoon almond flour
- 1 teaspoon organic baking powder
- Pinch of ground cinnamon
- 1 cup mozzarella cheese, shredded

Filling

- 2 tablespoons cream cheese, softened
- 2 tablespoons erythritol
- 1/4 teaspoon organic vanilla extract
- 2 fresh strawberries, hulled and chopped

Directions:

1. Preheat a mini waffle iron and then grease it.

2. For chaffles: in a bowl, add the egg and vanilla extract and mix well.

3. Add the flour, baking powder, and cinnamon, and mix until well combined.

4. Add the mozzarella cheese and stir to combine.

5. Place half of the mixture into preheated waffle iron and cook for about 4-minutes.

6. Repeat with the remaining mixture.

7. Meanwhile, for filling: in a bowl, place all the Ingredients: except the strawberry pieces and with a hand mixer, beat until well combined.

8. Serve each chaffle with cream cheese mixture and strawberry pieces.

Nutritional Values: Calories 143 Net Carb: g Total Fat 10.1 g Saturated Fat 4.5 g Cholesterol 100 mg Sodium 148 mg Total Carbs 4.1g Fiber 0.8 g Sugar 1.2 g Protein 7.6 g

49. Egg & Bacon Sandwich Chaffles

Servings: 4

Cooking Time: 20 Minutes

Ingredients:

Chaffles

- 2 large organic eggs, beaten
- 4 tablespoons almond flour
- 1 teaspoon organic baking powder
- 1 cup mozzarella cheese, shredded

Filling

- 4 organic fried eggs
- 4 cooked bacon slices

Directions:

1. Preheat a mini waffle iron and then grease it.

2. In a medium bowl, put all Ingredients: and with a fork, mix until well combined. Place half of the mixture into preheated waffle iron and cook for about 3-5 minutes.

3. Repeat with the remaining mixture.

4. Repeat with the remaining mixture.

5. Serve each chaffle with filling Ingredients.

Nutritional Values: Calories 197 Net Carb: g Total Fat 14.5 g Saturated Fat 4.1 g Cholesterol 2 mg Sodium 224 g Total Carbs 2.7 g Fiber 0.8 g Sugar 0.8 g Protein 12.9 g

50. Blueberry Peanut Butter Sandwich Chaffles

Servings: 2

Cooking Time: 10 minutes

Ingredients:

- 1 organic egg, beaten
- 1/2 cup cheddar cheese, shredded

Filling

- 2 tablespoons erythritol
- 1 tablespoon butter, softened
- 1 tablespoon natural peanut butter
- 2 tablespoons cream cheese, softened
- 1/4 teaspoon organic vanilla extract
- 2 teaspoons fresh blueberries

Directions:

1. Preheat a mini waffle iron and then grease it.

2. For chaffles: in a small bowl, add the egg and Cheddar cheese and stir to combine.

3. Place half of the mixture into preheated waffle iron and cook for about 5 minutes.

4. Repeat with the remaining mixture.

5. Meanwhile, for filling: In a medium bowl, put all Ingredients: and mix until well combined.

6. Serve each chaffle with peanut butter mixture.

Nutritional Values: Calories 143 Net Carbs 3.3 g Total Fat 10.1 g Saturated Fat 4.5 g Cholesterol 100 mg Sodium 148 mg Total Carbs 4.1g Fiber 0.8 g Sugar 1.2 g Protein 6 g

51. Chocolate Sandwich Chaffles

Servings: 2

Cooking Time: 10 minutes

Ingredients:

- Chaffles
- 1 organic egg, beaten
- 1 ounce cream cheese, softened
- 2 tablespoons almond flour
- 1 tablespoon cacao powder
- 2 teaspoons erythritol
- 1 teaspoon organic vanilla extract
- Filling
- 2 tablespoons cream cheese, softened
- 2 tablespoons erythritol
- 1/2 tablespoon cacao powder
- 1/4 teaspoon organic vanilla extract

Directions:

1. Preheat a mini waffle iron and then grease it.

2. For chaffles: In a medium bowl, put all Ingredients: and with a fork, mix until well combined. Place half of the mixture into preheated waffle iron and cook for about 3-5 minutes.

3. Repeat with the remaining mixture.

4. Meanwhile, for filling: In a medium bowl, put all Ingredients: and with a hand mixer, beat until well combined.

5. Serve each chaffle with chocolate mixture.

Nutritional Values: Calories 192 Net Carb: g Total Fat 16 g Saturated Fat 7.6 g Cholesterol 113 mg Sodium 115 mg Total Carbs 4.4 g Fiber 1.9 g Sugar 0.8 g Protein 5.7 g

52.   Berry Sauce Sandwich Chaffles

Servings: 2

Cooking Time: 8 Minutes

Ingredients:

- Filling
- 3 ounces frozen mixed berries,
- thawed with the juice
- 1 tablespoon erythritol
- 1 tablespoon water
- 1/4 tablespoon fresh lemon juice
- 2 teaspoons cream
- Chaffles
- 1 large organic egg, beaten
- 1/2 cup cheddar cheese, shredded
- 2 tablespoons almond flour

Directions:

1. For berry sauce: in a pan, add the berries, erythritol, water and lemon juice over medium heat and cook for about 8- minutes, pressing with the spoon occasionally.

2. Remove the pan of sauce from heat and set aside to cool before serving.

3. Preheat a mini waffle iron and then grease it.

4. In a bowl, add the egg, cheddar cheese and almond flour and beat until well combined. Place half of the mixture into preheated waffle iron and cook for about 3-5 minutes.

5. Repeat with the remaining mixture.

6. Serve each chaffle with cream and berry sauce.

Nutritional Values: Calories 222 Net Carbs 4.9 Total Fat 16 g Saturated Fat 7.2 g Cholesterol 123 mg Sodium 212 mg Total Carbs 7 g Fiber 2.3 g Sugar 3.8 g Protein 10.5 g

53.   Pork Sandwich Chaffles

Servings: 4

Cooking Time: 16 Minutes

Ingredients:

- Chaffles
- 2 large organic eggs
  11/4 cup superfine blanched almond flour
- 3/j teaspoon organic baking powder
- 1/2 teaspoon garlic powder
- 1 cup cheddar cheese, shredded
- Filling
- 12 ounces cooked pork, cut into slices
- 1 tomato, sliced
- 4 lettuce leaves

Directions:

1. Preheat a mini waffle iron and then grease it.

2. For chaffles: in a bowl, add the eggs, almond flour, baking powder, and garlic powder, and beat until well combined.

3. Add the cheese and stir to combine.

4. Place 1/4 of the mixture into preheated waffle iron and cook for about 3-minutes.

5. Repeat with the remaining mixture.

6. Serve each chaffle with filling Ingredients.

Nutritional Values: Calories 319 Net Carbs 2.5 g Total Fat 18.2 g Saturated Fat 8 g Cholesterol 185 mg Sodium 263 mg Total Carbs 3.5 g Fiber 1 g Sugar 0.g Protein 34.2 g

54. Tomato Sandwich Chaffles

Servings: 2

Cooking Time: 6 Minutes

Ingredients:

- Chaffles
- 1 large organic egg, beaten
- 1/2 cup of jack cheese, shredded
- finely
- 1/8 teaspoon organic vanilla extract
- Filling
- 1 small tomato, sliced
- 2 teaspoons fresh basil leaves

Directions:

1. Preheat a mini waffle iron and then grease it.

2. For chaffles: in a small bowl, place all the Ingredients: and stir to combine.

3. Place half of the mixture into preheated waffle iron and cook for about minutes.

4. Repeat with the remaining mixture.

5. Serve each chaffle with tomato slices and basil leaves.

Nutritional Values: Calories 155 Net Carbs 2.4 g Total Fat 11.g Saturated Fat 6.8 g Cholesterol 1i8 mg Sodium 217 mg Total Carbs 3 g Fiber 0.6 g Sugar 1.4 g Protein 9.6 g

55.   Salmon & Cream Sandwich Chaffles

Servings: 2

Cooking Time: 8 Minutes

Ingredients:

- Chaffles
- 1 organic egg, beaten
- 1/2 cup cheddar cheese, shredded
- 1 tablespoon almond flour
- 1 tablespoon fresh rosemary, chopped
- Filling
- 1/4 cup smoked salmon
- 1 teaspoon fresh dill, chopped
- 2 tablespoons cream

Directions:

1. Preheat a mini waffle iron and then grease it.

2. For chaffles: In a medium bowl, put all Ingredients: and with a fork, mix until well combined. Place half of the mixture into preheated waffle iron and cook for about 3-4 minutes.

3. Repeat with the remaining mixture.

4. Serve each chaffle with filling Ingredients.

Nutritional Values: Calories 202 Net Carbs 1.7 g Total Fat 11g Saturated Fat 7.5 g Cholesterol 118 mg Sodium 345 mg Total Carbs 2.9 g Fiber 1.2 g Sugar 0.7 g Protein 13.2 g

56.   Tuna Sandwich Chaffles

Servings: 2

Cooking Time: 8 Minutes

Ingredients:

Chaffles

- 1 organic egg, beaten
- 1/2 cup cheddar cheese, shredded
- 1 tablespoon almond flour
- Pinch of salt

Filling

- 1/4 cup water-packed tuna, flaked
- 2 lettuce leaves

Directions:

1. Preheat a mini waffle iron and then grease it.

2. For chaffles: In a medium bowl, put all Ingredients: and with a fork, mix until well combined. Place half of the mixture into preheated waffle iron and cook for about 3-4 minutes.

3. Repeat with the remaining mixture.

4. Serve each chaffle with filling Ingredients.

Nutritional Values: Calories 186 Net Carbs 0.9 g Total Fat 13.6 g Saturated Fat 6.8 g Cholesterol 120 mg Sodium 342 mg Total Carbs 1.3 g Fiber 0.4 g Sugar 0.g Protein 13.6 g

57. Easy Keto Chaffle Sausage Gravy

Servings: 2

Cooking Time: 10 Minutes

Ingredients:

For the Chaffle:

- 1 egg
- 1/2 cup mozzarella cheese, grated
- 1 tsp coconut flour
- 1 tsp water
- 1/4 tsp baking powder
- Pinch of salt

For the Keto Sausage Gravy:

- 1/4 cup breakfast sausage, browned
- 3 tbsp chicken broth
- 2 tbsp heavy whipping cream
- 2 tsp cream cheese, softened
- Dash garlic powder
- Pepper to taste
- Dash of onion powder (optional)

Directions:

1. Plug Dash Mini Waffle Maker into the wall and allow it to heat up. Grease lightly or use cooking spray.

2. Combine all the Ingredients: for the chaffle into a small bowl and stir to combine well.

3. Pour half of the chaffle batter onto

the waffle maker, then shut the lid and cook for approximately 4 minutes.

4. Remove chaffle from waffle maker and repeat the same process to make the second chaffle. Set aside to crisp.

5. For the Keto Sausage Gravy:

6. Cook one pound of breakfast sausage and drain. Reserve 1/4 cup for this.

7. Tip: Make sausage patties out of the rest of the sausage and reserve 1/4 a cup to brown for this. If you aren't familiar with breakfast sausage, it is crumbled like ground beef.

8. Wipe excess grease from the skillet and add 1/4 cup browned breakfast

sausage and the rest of the Ingredients: and bring to a boil stirring continuously.

9. Reduce heat to medium and continue to cook down with the lid off so that it begins to thicken for approx 5-7 minutes. If you1d like it very thick, you can add a bit of Xanthan Gum, but if you are patient with it simmering, the keto sausage gravy will thicken. Then, it will thicken even more as it cools.

10. Add salt and pepper to taste and spoon keto sausage gravy over chaffles.

11. Enjoy

Nutritional Values:(per serving):Calories: 2cal;Carbohydrates:3g; Protein: 11g;Fat: 17g;Saturated Fat:10 g;Cholesterol:134mg; Sodium:350 mg: Potassium: 133mg; Fiber: 1g; Sugar: 1g:Vitamin A: 595Iu;vitamin C: 2mg; Iron: I mg

58. Keto Chaffle Taco Shells

Servings: 5

Cooking Time: 20 Minutes

Ingredients:

- 1 tablespoon almond flour
- 1 cup taco blend cheese
- 2 eggs
- 1/4 tsp taco seasoning

Directions:

1. In a bowl, mix almond flour, taco blend cheese, eggs, and taco seasoning. I find it easiest to mix everything using a fork.

2. Add 1.5 tablespoons of taco chaffle batter to the waffle maker at a time — Cook chaffle batter in the waffle maker for 4 minutes.

3. Remove the taco chaffle shell from the waffle maker and drape over the side of a bowl. I used my pie pan because it was what I had on hand, but just about any bowl will work.

4. Continue making chaffle taco shells until you are out of batter. Then fill your taco shells with taco meat, your favorite TOPPINGs, and enjoy!

Nutritional Values:(per serving): Calories: 113kcal;Carbohydrates:1g;Protein: 8g;Fat: 99 ;Saturated Fat:4g ;Cholesterol:87mg; Sodium:181mg ; Potassium: 43mg;Fiber: 1g; Sugar: 1g ;Vitamin A: 243IU ;Calcium: 160mg; Iron: 1 mg

59.   Mini Keto Pizza Chaffle

Servings: 1

Cooking Time: 10 Minutes

Ingredients:

- 1/2 cup Shredded Mozzarella cheese
- 1 tablespoon almond flour
- 1/2 tsp baking powder
- 1 egg
- 1/4 tsp garlic powder
- 1/4 tsp basil
- 2 tablespoons low carb pasta sauce
- 2 tablespoons mozzarella cheese

Directions:

1. While the waffle maker is heating up, in a bowl mix mozzarella cheese, baking powder, garlic, basil, egg, and almond flour.

2. Pour i/the mixture into your mini waffle maker.

3. Cook for 5 minutes until your pizza waffle is completely cooked. If you check it and the waffle sticks to the waffle maker, let it cook for another minute or two.

4. Next, put the remainder of the pizza crust mix into the waffle maker and cook it.

5. Once both pizza crusts are cooked, place them on the baking sheet of your toaster oven.

6. Put 1 tablespoon of low carb pasta sauce on top of each pizza crust.

7. Sprinkle 1 tablespoon of shredded mozzarella cheese on top of each one.

8. Bake at 350 degrees in the toaster oven for roughly 5 minutes, just until the cheese is melted.

Nutritional Values:(per serving):Calories: 1kcal; Carbohydrates:4g; Protein: 139;Fat: 14g; Saturated Fat:6g; Cholesterol:116mg; Sodium:301m g: Potassium: 178mg; Fiber: 1g; Sugar: 1g: Vitamin A: 408IU;Calcium: 29omg;Iron: 1 mg

60.   Garlic Bread Chaffles

Servings: 2

Cooking Time: 11 Minutes

Ingredients:

- 1/2 cup shredded Mozzarella cheese
- 1 egg
- 1/2 tsp basil
- 1/4 tsp garlic powder
- 1 tbsp almond flour
- 1 tbsp butter
- 1/4 tsp garlic powder
- 1/4 cup shredded mozzarella cheese

Directions:

1. Heat up your Dash mini waffle maker.

2. In a small bowl, mix the egg, 1/tsp basil, l/1j tsp garlic powder, 1 tablespoon almond flour and ½ cup Mozzarella Cheese.

3. Add 1/2 of the batter into your mini waffle maker and cook for 4 minutes. If they are still a bit uncooked, leave it cooking for another 2 minutes. Then cook the rest of the batter to make a second chaffle.

4. In a small bowl, add tablespoon butter and 1/tsp garlic powder and melt in the microwave. It will take about 25 seconds or so, depending on your microwave.

5. Place the chaffles on a baking sheet and use a rubber brush to spread the butter and garlic mixture on top.

6. Add i/8th a cup of cheese on top of each chaffle.

7. Put chaffles in the oven or a toaster oven at 400 degrees and cook until the cheese is melted.

Nutritional Values:(per serving): Calories: 231kcal ;Carbohydrates:2g ;Protein: 139;Fat: 19g ;Saturated Fat:l0g ;Cholesterol:130mg ;Sodium:346mg ; Potassium: 52mg ; Fiber: 1g ;Sugar: 1g ;Vitamin A: 5IU ;Calcium: 232mg ;Iron: I mg

51.   Basic Keto Low Carb Chaffle

Servings: 1

Cooking Time: 8 Minutes

Ingredients:

- 1 egg
- 1/2 cup cheddar cheese, shredded

Direction:

1. Turn waffle maker on or plug it in so that it heats and grease both sides.

2. In a small bowl, crack an egg, then add the i/cup cheddar cheese and stir to combine.

3. Pour 1/2 of the batter in the waffle maker and close the top.

4. Cook for 3-minutes or until it reaches desired doneness.

5. Carefully remove from waffle maker and set aside for 2-3 minutes to give it time to crisp.

6. Follow the Directions: again to make the second chaffle.

Nutritional Values:(per serving):Calories 291kcal;Carbohydrates:lg;Protein: 2og;Fat 23g;Saturated Fat:13g;Cholesterol:223mg;Sodium:41₃ mg: Potassium: 116mg;Sugar: ig:Vitamin A 804Iu;Calcium: 432mg;lron: 1mg

62.   Chaffle Keto Protein Chaffle

Servings: 1

Cooking Time: 8 Minutes

Ingredients:

- 1 egg (beaten)
- 1/2 cup whey protein powder
- A pinch of salt
- 1 tsp baking powder
- 3 tbsp sour cream
- 1/2 tsp vanilla extract

TOPPING:

- 2 tbsp heavy cream
- 1 tbsp granulated swerve

Directions:

1. Plug the waffle maker to preheat it and spray it with a non-stick cooking spray.

2. In a mixing bowl, whisk together the egg, vanilla and sour cream.

3. In another mixing bowl, combine the protein powder, baking powder and salt.

4. Pour the flour mixture into the egg mixture and mix until the Ingredients: are well combined and you form a smooth batter.

5. Pour an appropriate amount of the batter into the waffle maker and spread the batter to the edges to cover all the holes on the waffle maker.

6. Close the waffle maker and cook for about 4 minutes or according to your waffle maker's settings.

7. After the cooking cycle, use a plastic or silicone utensil to remove the chaffle from the waffle iron.

8. Repeat step 4 to 6 until you have cooked all the batter into chaffles.

9. For the TOPPING, whisk together the cream and swerve in a mixing bowl until smooth and fluffy.

10. Top the chaffles with the cream and enjoy.

Nutritional Values: Per Servings: Fat 25.9g 33% Carbohydrate 13.1g 5% Sugars 2.1g Protein 41.6g

63.   Chaffle Tacos

Servings: 4

Cooking Time: 15 Minutes

Ingredients:

- Chaffle:
- 2 tbsp coconut flour
- 3 eggs (beaten)
- 1/2 cup shredded mozzarella cheese
- 1/2 cup shredded cheddar cheese
- A pinch of salt
- 1/2 tsp oregano
- Taco Filling:
- 1 garlic clove (minced)
- 1 small onion (finely chopped)
- 1/2 pound ground beef
- 1 tsp olive oil
- 1 tsp cumin
- 1/2 tsp Italian seasoning
- 1 tsp paprika
- 1 tsp chili powder
- 1 tomato (diced)
- 1 green bell pepper (diced)
- 4 tbsp sour cream

- 1 tbsp chopped green onions

Directions:

1. Plug the waffle maker to preheat it and spray it with a non-stick cooking spray.

2. In a mixing bowl, combine the mozzarella cheese, cheddar, coconut flour, salt and oregano. Add the eggs and mix until the Ingredients: are well combined.

3. Fill the waffle maker with an appropriate amount of the batter. Spread the batter to the edges to cover all the hole on the waffle maker.

4. Close the waffle maker and cook for about 5 minutes or according to waffle maker's settings.

5. After the cooking cycle, use a plastic

or silicone utensil to remove the chaffle from the waffle maker. Set aside.

6. Repeat step 3 to 5 until you have cooked all the batter into chaffles.

7. Heat up a large skillet over medium to high heat.

8. Add the ground beef and saute until it is browned, breaking it apart while sauteing. Transfer the beef to a paper towel lined plate to drain and wipe the skillet clean.

9. Add the olive oil and leave it to get hot.

10. Add the onions and garlic and saute for 3-4 minutes or until the onion is translucent, stirring often.

11. Add the diced tomatoes and green pepper. Cook for 1 minute.

12. Add the browned ground beef. Stir in the cumin, paprika, chili powder and Italian seasoning.

13. Reduce the heat and cook on low for about 8 minutes, stirring often to prevent burning.

14. Remove the skillet from heat.

15. Scoop the taco mixture into the chaffles and top with chopped green onion and sour cream.

16. Enjoy.

Nutritional Values: Per Servings: Fat 59 22% Carbohydrate 12.6g 5% Sugars 4.59 Protein 28.6g

64.   Chaffle With Sausage Gravy

Servings: 2

Cooking Time: 15 Minutes

Ingredients:

- Sausage Gravy:
- 1/4 cup cooked breakfast sausage
- 1/8 tsp onion powder
- 1/8 tsp garlic powder
- 1/2 tsp pepper or more to taste
- 3 tbsp chicken broth
- 2 tsp cream cheese
- 2 tbsp heavy whipping cream
- 1/4 tsp oregano
- Chaffle:
- 1 tbsp almond flour
- 1 tbsp finely chopped onion
- 1/8 tsp salt
- 1/4 tsp baking powder
- 1/2 cup mozzarella cheese
- 1 egg (beaten)

Directions:

1. Plug the waffle maker to preheat it and spray it with a non-stick spray.

2. In a mixing bowl, combine the almond flour, chopped onion, mozzarella, baking powder and salt. Add the egg and mix until the Ingredients: are well combined.

3. Fill the waffle maker with 1/2 of the batter and spread the batter to the edges to cover all the holes on the waffle maker.

4. Close the waffle maker and bake for about minutes or according to waffle maker's settings.

5. After the baking cycle, remove the chaffle from the waffle maker with a silicone or plastic utensil.

6. Repeat step 3 to 5 until you have cooked all the batter into chaffles.

7. Heat up a skillet over medium to high heat. Add cooked sausage and sear until the sausage is browned, stirring often to prevent burning.

8. Pour in the chicken broth and add the oregano, garlic powder, onion powder, pepper, cream cheese and whipping cream.

9. Bring to a boil, reduce the heat and simmer for about 7 minutes or until the gravy sauce thickens.

10. Serve the chaffles with the gravy and enjoy.

Nutritional Values: Per Servings: Fat 16.6g 21% Carbohydrate 3.39 1% Sugars 0.7g Protein 9.8g

65. Lettuce Chaffle Sandwich

Servings: 2

Cooking Time: 5 Minutes

Ingredients:

- 1 large egg
- 1 tbsp. almond flour
- 1 tbsp. full-fat Greek yogurt
- 1/8 tsp baking powder
- 1/4 cup shredded Swiss cheese " 4 lettuce leaves

Directions:

1. Switch on your waffle maker.

2. Grease it with cooking spray.

3. Mix together egg, almond flour, yogurts, baking powder and cheese in mixing bowl.

4. Pour 1/2 cup of the batter into the center of your waffle iron and close the lid.

5. Cook chaffles for about 2-3 minutes until cooked through.

6. Repeat with remaining batter

7. Once cooked, carefully transfer to plate. Serve lettuce leaves between 2 chaffles.

8. Enjoy!

Nutritional Values: Per Servings: Protein: 22% 4o kcal Fat: 66% 120 kcal Carbohydrates: 12% 22 kcal

56.   Shrimp Avocado Chaffle Sandwich

Servings: 4

Cooking Time: 32 Minutes

Ingredients:

- 2 cups shredded mozzarella cheese
- 4 large eggs
- 1/2 tsp curry powder
- 1/2 tsp oregano
- Shrimp Sandwich Filling:
- 1-pound raw shrimp (peeled and deveined)
- 1 large avocado (diced)
- 4 slices cooked bacon
- 2 tbsp sour cream
- 1/2 tsp paprika
- 1 tsp Cajun seasoning
- 1 tbsp olive oil
- 1/4 cup onion (finely chopped)
- 1 red bell pepper (diced)

Directions:

1. Plug the waffle maker to preheat it and spray it with a non-stick cooking spray.

2. Break the eggs into a mixing bowl and beat. Add the cheese, oregano and curry. Mix until the Ingredients: are well combined.

3. Pour an appropriate amount of the batter into the waffle maker and spread out the batter to the edges to cover all the holes on the waffle maker. This should make 8 mini waffles.

4. Close the waffle maker and cook for about minutes or according to your waffle maker's settings.

5. After the cooking cycle, use a silicone or plastic utensil to remove the chaffle from the waffle maker.

6. Repeat step 3 to 5 until you have cooked all the batter into chaffles.

7. Heat up the olive oil in a large skillet over medium to high heat.

8. Add the shrimp and cook until the shrimp is pink and tender.

9. Remove the skillet from heat and use a slotted spoon to transfer the shrimp to a paper towel lined plate to drain for a few minutes.

10. Put the shrimp in a mixing bowl. Add paprika and Cajun seasoning. Toss until the shrimps are all coated with seasoning.

11. To assemble the sandwich, place one chaffle on a flat surface and spread some sour cream over it. Layer some shrimp, onion, avocado, diced pepper and one slice of bacon over it. Cover with another chaffle.

12. Repeat step 10 until you have assembled all the Ingredients: into sandwiches.

13. Serve and enjoy.

Nutritional Values: Per Servings: Fat 32.1g 41% Carbohydrate io.8g 4% Sugars 2.5g Protein 44.8g

67.   Cuban Pork Sandwich

Servings: 1

Cooking Time: 10 Minutes

Ingredients:

- Sandwich Filling:
- 25 g swiss cheese (sliced)
- 2 ounces cooked deli ham (thinly sliced)
- 3 slices pickle chips
- 1/2 tbsp Dijon mustard
- 1/2 tbsp mayonnaise
- 3 ounces pork roast
- 1 tsp paprika
- 1 stalk celery (diced)
- Chaffle:
- 1 tsp baking powder
- 1 large egg (beaten)
- 1 tbsp full-fat Greek yogurt
- 4 tbsp mozzarella cheese
- 1 tbsp almond flour

Directions:

1. Preheat the oven to 350°F and grease a baking sheet.

2. Plug the waffle maker to preheat it and spray it with a non-stick cooking spray.

3. In a mixing bowl, combine the almond flour, cheese and baking powder.

4. Add the egg and yogurt. Mix until the Ingredients: are well combined.

5. Fill the waffle maker with an appropriate amount of the batter and spread the batter to the edges to cover all the holes on the waffle maker.

6. Close the waffle maker and cook the waffle until it is crispy. That will take about 5 minutes. The time may vary in some waffle makers.

7. After the cooking cycle, remove the chaffle from the waffle maker with a plastic or silicone utensil.

8. Repeat step 4 to 6 until you have cooked all the batter into chaffles.

9. In a small mixing bowl, combine the mustard, oregano and mayonnaise.

10. Brush the mustard-mayonnaise mixture over the surface of both chaffles.

11. Layer the pork, ham, pickles and celery over one of the chaffles. Layer the cheese slices on top and cover it with the second chaffle.

12. Place it on the baking sheet. Place it in oven and bake until the cheese melts. You can place a heavy stainless place over the chaffle to make the sandwich come out flat after baking

13. After the baking cycle, remove the chaffle sandwich from the oven and let it cool for a few minutes.

14. Serve warm and enjoy.

Nutritional Values: Per Servings: Fat 52.3g 67% Carbohydrate 17.3g 6% Sugars 2.7g Protein 82.6g

58. Tuna Salad Chaffles

Servings: 2

Cooking Time: 8 Minutes

Ingredients:

Tuna Sandwich:

- 1 can water packed tuna (drained)
- 1 small sweet onion (chopped)
- 1 green bell pepper (finely chopped)
- 1 small carrot (peeled and chopped)
- 2 tbsp mayonnaise
- 1/2 tsp paprika
- 1/4 tsp ground black pepper or to taste
- 1/4 tsp salt or to taste
- 1 celery stalk (chopped)
- 1 tbsp freshly chopped parsley

Chaffle:

- 2 eggs (beaten)
- 4 tbsp almond flour
- 1 cup shredded mozzarella cheese
- 1/4 tsp baking powder
- 1/2 tsp garlic powder

Directions:

1. Plug the waffle maker to preheat it and spray the it with a non-stick cooking spray.

2. In a mixing bowl, combine the almond flour, baking powder, garlic powder and mozzarella. Add the eggs and mix until the Ingredients: are well combined.

3. Fill the waffle maker with an appropriate amount of the batter and spread the batter to the edges to cover all the holes on the waffle maker.

4. Close the waffle maker and cook for about minutes or according to waffle maker's settings.

5. After the cooking cycle, use a silicone or plastic utensil to remove the chaffle from the waffle maker.

6. Repeat step 3 to 5 until you have cooked all the batter into chaffles.

7. In a mixing bowl, combine the tuna, celery, pepper, onion, salt, paprika, carrot, onion and green pepper. Add the mayonnaise and toss until the Ingredients: are well combined.

8. Place one of the chaffle of a flat surface and spoon 1/2 of the tuna salad into it. Top with fresh parsley. Cover it with another chaffle and press.

9. Repeat step 8 to make the second sandwich.

10. Serve and enjoy.

Nutritional Values: Per Servings: Fat 26.3g 34% Carbohydrate 1g.6g 7% Sugars 7.79 Protein 37.8g

69. Keto Pizza Chaffe

Servings: 2

Cooking Time: 15 Minutes

Ingredients:

Pizza Filing:

- 1/3 cups pepperoni slices
- 1 tbsp marinara sauce
- 1/2 cup shredded mozzarella cheese
- 1 onion (finely chopped)
- 1 small green bell pepper (finely chopped)

Chaffle:

- 1 egg (beaten)
- A pinch of Italian seasoning
- A pinch of salt
- 1/2 cup mozzarella cheese
- 1/4 tsp baking powder
- 1/2 tsp dried basil
- A pinch of garlic powder
- 1 tbsp + 1tsp almond flour

Directions:

1. Preheat the oven to 400°F and line a baking sheet with parchment paper.

2. Plug the waffle maker and preheat it. Spray it with a nonstick spray.

3. For the chaffle: In a mixing bowl, combine the baking powder, almond flour, garlic powder, Italian seasoning, basil, mozzarella cheese and salt. Add the egg and mix until the Ingredients: are well combined.

4. Fill the waffle maker with appropriate amount of the batter and spread the batter to the edges of the waffle maker to cover all the holes on the waffle maker.

5. Close the lid of the waffle maker and cook for about minutes or according to waffle maker's settings.

6. After the baking cycle, remove the chaffle from waffle maker with a silicone or plastic utensil.

7. Repeat step 4 to 6 until you have cooked all the batter into chaffles.

8. Top each of the chaffles with the marinara sauce, sprinkle the finely chopped onions and pepper over the chaffles.

9. Top with shredded mozzarella cheese and layer the pepperoni slices on the cheese TOPPING.

10. Gently place the chaffles on the lined baking sheet. Place the baking sheet in the oven and bake for about 5 minutes. Afterwards, broil for about 1 minute.

11. Remove the pizza chaffles from the oven and let them cook for a few minutes.

12. Serve warm and enjoy.

Nutritional Values: Per Servings: Fat 23.2g 30% Carbohydrate 14.9g 5% Sugars 6.8g Protein 16.8g

70.   Cauliflower Turkey Chaffle

Servings: 2

Cooking Time: 12 Minutes

Ingredients:

- 1 large egg (beaten)
- 1/2 cup cauliflower rice
- 1/4 cup diced turkey
- 1/2 tsp coconut aminos or soy sauce
- A pinch of ground black pepper
- A pinch of white pepper
- 1/4 tsp curry
- 1/4 tsp oregano
- 1 tbsp butter (melted)
- 3/j cup shredded mozzarella cheese
- 1 garlic clove (crushed)

Directions:

1. Plug the waffle maker to preheat it and spray it with a non-stick spray.

2. In a mixing bowl, combine the cauliflower rice, white pepper, black pepper, curry and oregano.

3. In another mixing bowl, whisk together the eggs, butter, crushed garlic and coconut aminos.

4. Pour the egg mixture into the cheese mixture and mix until the Ingredients: are well combined.

5. Add the diced turkey and stir to combine.

6. Sprinkle 2 tbsp cheese over the waffle maker. Fill the waffle maker with an appropriate amount of the batter. Spread out the batter to the edges to cover all the holes on the waffle maker. Sprinkle another 2 tbsp cheese over the batter.

7. Close the waffle maker and cook for about 4 minutes or according to waffle maker's settings.

8. After the cooking cycle, use a plastic or silicone utensil to remove the chaffle from the waffle maker.

9. Repeat step 6 to 8 until you have cooked all the batter into chaffles.

10. Serve warm and enjoy.

Nutritional Values: Per Servings: Fat 5g15% Carbohydrate 3.8g 1% Sugars 1.2g Protein 12.5g

71. Pork Chaffles On Pan

Servings: 4

Cooking Time: 5 minutes

Ingredients:

- 1 cup pork, minced
- 1 tsp cream cheese

TOPPING:

- Sour cream

Directions:

1. Plug the waffle maker to preheat it and spray it with a non-stick spray.

2. In a mixing bowl, combine parmesan, cheddar, jalapeno, salt, ground pepper, garlic powder and onion powder.

3. Whisk together the egg and cream cheese. Pour it into the cheese mixture and mix until the Ingredients: are well combined. Fold in the diced chicken.

4. Fill the waffle maker with about 1/2 of the batter and spread out the batter to cover all the holes on the waffle maker.

5. Close the waffle maker and cook for about minutes or according to waffle maker's settings.

6. After the cooking cycle, use a plastic or silicone utensi to remove the chaffle from the waffle maker.

7. Repeat step 4 to 6 until the you have cooked all the batter into chaffles.

8. Serve warm and top with sour cream as desired.

Nutritional Values: Per Servings: Fat 13.4g 17% Carbohydrate 1.3g 0% Sugars 0.6g Protein 46.3

72.   Savory Chaffles

Servings: 4

Cooking Time: 5minutes

Ingredients:

- 1 egg
- 1 cup cheddar cheese
- pinch of salt
- 2 green chilies, chopped
- 1 tsp. red chilly flakes
- 1/2 cup spinach chopped
- 1/2 cup cauliflower
- 1 pinch garlic powder
- 1 pinch onion powder
- 1 tbsp. coconut oil

Directions:

1. Heat your nonstick pan over medium heat.

2. Blend all Ingredients: except oil in a blender.

3. Grease pan with avocado oil.

4. Once the pan is hot, pour 2 tbsps. cauliflower batter and cook for about 1-2 minutes

5. Flip and cook for another 1-2 minutes

6. Once chaffle is brown, remove from pan.

7. Serve hot and enjoy!

Nutritional Values: Per Servings: Protein: 32% 42 kcal
Fat: 63% kcal Carbohydrates: 5% 6 kcal

73. Oven-baked Chaffles

Servings: 10

Cooking Time: 5 Minutes

Ingredients:

- 3 eggs
- 2 cups mozzarella cheese
- 1/4 cup coconut flour
- 1 tsp. baking powder
- 1 tbsp. coconut oil
- 1 tsp stevia
- 1 tbsp. coconut cream

Directions:

1. Preheat oven on 400 F.

2. Mix together all Ingredients: in a bowl.

3. Pour batter in silicon waffle mold and set it on a baking tray.

4. Bake chaffles in an oven for about

10-15 minutes

5. Once cooked, remove from oven

6. Serve hot with coffee and enjoy!

Nutritional Values: Per Servings: Protein: 34% 3kcal Fat
61% 66 kcal Carbohydrates: 5% 6 kcal

74.   Buffalo Chicken Chaffle

Servings: 2

Cooking Time: 10 Minutes

Ingredients:

- 1 egg
- 5 ounces cooked chicken (diced)
- 2 tbsp buffalo sauce
- 12 tsp garlic powder
- 1/2 tsp onion powder
- 1/2 tsp dried basil
- 5 tbsp shredded cheddar cheese
- 2 ounces cream cheese

Directions:

1. Plug the waffle maker and preheat it. Spray it with non-stick spray.

2. In a large mixing bowl, combine the onion powder, basil, garlic, buffalo sauce, cheddar cheese chicken and cream cheese. Mix until the Ingredients: are well combined and you have formed a smooth batter.

3. Sprinkle some shredded cheddar cheese over the waffle maker and pour in adequate amount of the batter.

Spread out the batter to the edges of the waffle maker to cover al the holes on the waffle maker.

4. Close the lid of the waffle maker and cook for about 3 to minutes or according to waffle maker's settings.

5. After the cooking cycle, remove the chaffle from the waffle maker with a plastic or silicone utensil.

6. Repeat step 3 to 5 until you have cooked all the batter into chaffles.

7. Serve and enjoy.

Nutritional Values: Per Servings: Fat 20.lg 26% Carbohydrate 2.2g 1% Sugars 0.7g Protein 30g

75. Sloppy Joe Chaffle

Servings: 2

Cooking Time: 20 Minutes

Ingredients:

Chaffle:

- 1 large egg (beaten)
- 1/8 tsp onion powder
- 1 tbsp almond flour
- 1/2 cup shredded mozzarella cheese
- 1 tsp nutmeg
- 1/4 tsp baking powder

Sloppy Joe Filling:

- 2 tsp olive oil
- 1 pounds ground beef
- 1 celery stalk (chopped)
- 2 tbsp ketch up
- 2 tsp Worcestershire sauce
- 1 small onions (chopped)
- 1 green bell pepper (chopped)
- 1 tbsp sugar free maple syrup
- 1 cup tomato sauce (7.9 ounce)
- 2 garlic cloves (minced)

- 1/2 tsp salt or to taste
- 1/2 tsp ground black pepper or to taste

Directions:

1. For the chaffle:

2. Plug the waffle maker and preheat it. Spray it with non-stick spray.

3. Combine the baking powder, nutmeg, flour and onion powder in a mixing bowl. Add the eggs and mix.

4. Add the cheese and mix until the Ingredients: are well combined and you have formed a smooth batter.

5. Pour the batter into the waffle maker and spread it out to the edges of the waffle maker to cover all the holes on it.

6. Close the waffle lid and cook for about 5 minutes or according to waffle maker's settings.

7. After the cooking cycle, remove the chaffle from the waffle maker with a plastic or silicone utensil. Transfer the chaffle to a wire rack to cool.

8. For the sloppy joe Ming:

9. Heat up a large skillet over medium to high heat.

10. Add the ground beef and saute until the beef is browned.

11. Use a slotted spoon to transfer the ground beef to a paper towel lined plate to drain. Drain all the grease in the skillet.

12. Add the olive oil to the skillet and heat it up.

13. Add the onions, green pepper, celery and garlic. Saute until the veggies are tender, stirring often to prevent burning.

14. Stir in the tomato sauce, Worcestershire sauce, ketchup, maple syrup, salt and pepper.

15. Add the browned beef and bring the mixture to a boil. Reduce the heat and simmer for about 10 minutes.

16. Remove the skillet from heat.

17. Scoop the sloppy joe into the chaffles and enjoy.

Nutritional Values: Per Servings: Fat 30.5g 39% Carbohydrate 26.2g 10% Sugars 15.3g Protein 80.2g

76. Chaffle And Cheese Sandwich

Servings: 3

Cooking Time: 5 minutes

Ingredients:

- 1 egg
- 1/2 cup mozzarella cheese
- 1 tsp. baking powder
- 3 slice feta cheese for TOPPING

Directions:

1. Make 6 chaffles

2. Set feta cheese between two chaffles.

3. Serve with hot coffee and enjoy!

Nutritional Values: Per Servings: Protein: 31% 56 kcal Fat: 60% no kcal Carbohydrates: g% 16 kcal

77.   Chicken Parmesan Chaffle

Servings: 2

Cooking Time: 13 Minutes

Ingredients:

- 1 egg (beaten)
- 1/2 cup shredded chicken
- 2 tbsp shredded parmesan cheese
- 1/3 cup shredded mozzarella cheese
- 1/4 tsp garlic powder
- 1/4 tsp onion powder
- 2 tbsp marinara sauce
- 1 tsp Italian seasoning
- Garnish:
- 1 tbsp chopped green onions

Directions:

1. Plug the waffle maker to preheat it and spray it with a non-stick cooking spray.

2. In a mixing bowl, combine the mozzarella cheese, shredded chicken, Italian seasoning, onion powder and garlic powder. Add the egg and mix until the Ingredients: are well combined.

3. Pour half of the batter into the

waffle maker and spread out the batter to the edges to cover all the holes on the waffle maker.

4. Close the waffle maker and cook for about minutes or according to your waffle maker's settings.

5. Meanwhile, preheat your oven to 400°F and line a baking sheet with parchment paper.

6. After the cooking cycle, use a plastic or silicone utensil to remove the chaffle from the waffle maker.

7. Repeat 3, 4 and 6 to make the second chaffle.

8. Spread marinara sauce over the surface of both chaffles and sprinkle the parmesan cheese over the chaffles.

9. Arrange the chaffles into the baking

sheet and place them in the oven. Bake for about 5 minutes or until the cheese melts.

10. Remove the chaffles from the oven and let them cool for a few minutes.

11. Serve and top with chopped green onion.

Nutritional Values: Per Servings: Fat 6.7g g% Carbohydrate 3.79 1% Sugars 2g Protein 16.9g

78.   Lobster Chaffle

Servings: 2

Cooking Time: 8 Minutes

Ingredients:

- 1 egg (beaten)
- 1/2 cup shredded mozzarella cheese
- 1/4 tsp garlic powder
- 1/4 tsp onion powder
- 1/8 tsp Italian seasoning
- Lobster Filling:
- 1/2 cup lobster tails (defrosted)
- 1 tbsp mayonnaise
- 1 tsp dried basil
- 1 tsp lemon juice
- 1 tbsp chopped green onion

Directions:

1. Plug the waffle maker to preheat it and spray it with a non-stick cooking spray.

2. In a mixing bowl, combine the mozzarella, Italian seasoning, garlic and onion powder. Add the egg and mix until the Ingredients: are well combined.

3. Pour an appropriate amount of the batter into the waffle maker and spread out the batter to cover all the holes on the waffle maker.

4. Close the waffle maker and cook for about minutes or according to your waffle maker's settings.

5. After the cooking cycle, use a plastic or silicone utensil to remove and transfer the chaffle to a wire rack to cool.

6. Repeat step 3 to 5 until you have cooked all the batter into chaffles.

7. For the filling, put the lobster tail in a mixing bowl and add the mayonnaise, basil and lemon juice. Toss until the Ingredients: are well combine.

8. Fill the chaffles with the lobster mixture and garnish with chopped green onion.

9. Serve and enjoy.

Nutritional Values: Per Servings : Fat 6.3g 8% Carbohydrate 39 1% Sugars 1g Protein n.gg

79. Broccoli Chaffles On Pan

Servings: 4

Cooking Time: 5 Minutes

Ingredients:

- 1 egg
- 1 cup cheddar cheese
- 1/2 cup broccoli chopped
- 1 tsp baking powder
- 1 pinch garlic powder
- 1 pinch salt
- 1 pinch black pepper
- 1 tbsp. coconut oil

Directions:

1. Heat your nonstick pan over medium heat.

2. Mix together all Ingredients: in a bowl.

3. Grease pan with oil.

4. Once the pan is hot, pour broccoli and cheese batter on greased pan

5. Cook for 1-2 minutes.

6. Flip and cook for another 1-2 minutes.

7. Once chaffles are brown, remove from the pan.

8. Serve with raspberries and melted coconut oil on top.

9. Enjoy!

Nutritional Values: Per Servings :Protein: 20% 40 kca
Fat: 72% 142 kcal Carbohydrates: 7% 15 kcal

80. Chicken Chaffles With Tzatziki

Servings: 2

Cooking Time: 12 Minutes

Ingredients:

- Chaffles

  - 1 organic egg, beaten
  - 1/3 cup grass-fed cooked chicken, chopped
  - 1/3 cup mozzarella cheese, shredded
  - 1/4 teaspoon garlic, minced
  - 1/4 teaspoon dried basil, crushed
  - Tzatziki
  - 1/4 cup plain Greek yogurt
  - 1/2 of small cucumber, peeled, seeded, and chopped
  - 1 teaspoon olive oil
  - 1/2 teaspoon fresh lemon juice
  - Pinch of ground black pepper
  - 1/4 tablespoon fresh dill, chopped
  - 1/2 of garlic clove, peeled

Directions:

1. Preheat a mini waffle iron and then grease it.

2. For chaffles: In a medium bowl, put all Ingredients: and with your hands, mix until well combined. Place half of the mixture into preheated waffle iron and cook for about 4-6 minutes.

3. Repeat with the remaining mixture.

4. Meanwhile, for tzatziki: in a food processor, place all the Ingredients: and pulse until well combined.

5. Serve warm chaffles alongside the tzatziki.

Nutritional Values: Calories 131 Net Carbs 4.4 g Total Fat 5 g Saturated Fat 2 g Cholesterol 104 mg Sodium 97 mg Total Carbs 4.7 g Fiber O.3 g Sugar 3 g Protein 13 g

81. Savory Pork Rind Chaffle

Servings: 2

Cooking Time: 10 Minutes

Ingredients:

- 1/4 tsp paprika
- 1/4 tsp oregano
- 1/4 tsp garlic powder
- 1/8 tsp ground black pepper or to taste
- 1/2 onion (finely chopped)
- 1/2 cup pork rind (crushed)
- 1/2 cup mozzarella cheese
- 1 large egg (beaten)

Directions:

1. Plug the waffle maker to preheat it and spray with a non-stick cooking spray.

2. In a mixing bowl, combine the crushed pork rind, cheese, onion, paprika, garlic powder and pepper. Add the egg and mix until the Ingredients: are well combined.

3. Pour an appropriate amount of the batter into the waffle maker and spread out the batter to cover all the holes on the waffle maker.

4. Close the waffle maker and cook for about 5 minutes or according to your waffle maker's settings.

5. After the cooking cycle, use a plastic or silicone utensil to remove the chaffle from the waffle maker.

6. Repeat step 3 to 5 until you have cooked all the batter into chaffles.

7. Serve and top with sour cream as desired.

Nutritional Values: Per Servings : Fat 24g 31% Carbohydrate 3.6g 1% Sugars 1.5g Protein 41.9g

CONCLUSIONS

THE KETOGENIC DIET

The Ketogenic Diet or 'Keto', as you may have heard, primarily revolves around the cut down of carbohydrates. It consists of foods containing high fat and very low carbohydrates along with moderate helpings of protein. If you wish to get into the nitty-gritty of it, in a 2000 kcal per day diet, the carbohydrates intake would be limited to 20 to 50 g per day.

This particular and rather steep reduction pushes the body into a metabolic state known as 'ketosis' hence the name 'keto.' When this occurs, the body becomes efficient in burning down fat in the body to produce energy for bodily function and brain activity. This is because, normally, carbohydrates are the primary source of energy to the body. So, when that intake seizes, the body automatically switches to alternative means i.e. burning down fats in your body for energy.

While the masses switch to Ketogenic Diet for weight loss purposes and losing a few inches on the scale. It may be beneficial to note that this diet was first introduced by Russel Wilder while trying to treat patients with epilepsy.

- KETO LIFESTYLE

There are a profound number of diets out there in the world. Some of them are quite effective, and yet some are only successful in making you starve. Of all the diet advice that you have come upon, you must surely have heard that the only time a diet truly works is when you are consistent in your work and turn it into a lifestyle. This holds true in all cases, especially the Keto diet.

The truth of the matter is, that while a Keto diet will give you short-term benefits such as increased energy and reduced body weight, you may fall back into your unhealthy lifestyle quite easily. This is one of the many reasons why it is essential to adopt Keto as not only your diet but as a lifestyle as well.

There is only one remaining question now: What will it take to fall into the Keto lifestyle?

Well, one of the obvious answers would be to firstly give more depth and meaning to your diet. Weight loss should not be the only viable reason you follow it.

Weight loss can be achieved with any diet. However, the root issue always presents itself in the end: These diets eventually fail. The reason for this is that those diets do not balance your hormones, due to which you are always

178

hungry. And, of course, it becomes extremely difficult to follow a diet when you get constant hunger pangs.

It is also important to note that once the target weight is achieved, the motivation to continue is lost, and, once again, you fall back into the same pattern and routine.

Our point is: It will do you well to give more dimensions to your diet journey than just to lose weight.

It is vital to have integral knowledge of what a Keto lifestyle entails and of what are the long-term benefits other than just the physical ones.

Once your body is in the Ketosis metabolic state, it starts using ketone as a source of energy. This, along with promoting fat loss, also helps in increasing your energy, balancing your hormones, and lowering your cholesterol levels.

Moreover, Keto diet has been linked to improving glucose levels, increased concentration levels, improved mental health, reduced appetite, and reduced inflammation.

It is a well-known fact that saturated fats are not that popular. However, a balanced diet that contains good quality fats has profound health benefits.

One thing that can help you follow the Keto lifestyle is stocking your kitchen full of healthy Keto substitutes. This will not only help you avoid unnecessary sugars, but it is a foolproof way to make sure you don't end up giving in to unhealthy cravings all the time.

And the bonus is: A Keto diet tastes just as good as your normal everyday diet!

One other trick that can help you follow this lifestyle is having a support group. Support and accountability go a long way in helping you follow the right track and makes a significant difference in how often you transgress from it.

Lastly, it would do you well to have meal plans, which not only help you in taking in more nutrients, but they make it easier to follow. To add to the benefits, even if meal plans are time taking at first, this can also save you plenty of time in the long-run if you include meal preps in your plans. Less food will go to waste because of which you can even save money.

All you have to do is pick out some of your favorite Keto recipes and circle them throughout the week.

The key to reaping all the benefits of Keto diet is to make it a permanent lifestyle, and it can be done quite easily just by following the simple steps that we have mentioned above.

- ## WHY CHOOSE KETOGENIC DIET?

The Ketogenic Diet is known to do a lot more than just aid weight loss. Other benefits include a lower risk of heart disease as the less carbohydrate you intake, the more fat in your body gets broken down to produce energy. The whole process in turn, allows your body to feel energetic as compared to when you eat a lot of carbs and end up feeling bloated and sluggish. Diet followers have in fact, reported back, claiming they are more energetic and thus active around the home.

All the meals in a ketogenic diet are made in olive oil. Sugar is replaced with natural sweeteners and is derived from plants, thus making them a hundred percent diabetic-friendly. Flour is replaced with almond or coconut flour which in turn have numerous health benefits on their own. And setting all that aside, you get to eat as much cheese as you could possibly like- I mean, what more do you want?

Another major perk of the Ketogenic Diet is workouts are not particularly necessary as they are when it comes to other diets. Thus, not many lifestyle changes are required when switching to keto-friendly meals.

Ketogenic Diet when done right with an array of vegetables, proteins, and vitamins, can enable you to sleep better, function proactively, and even tackle hair loss!

- TIME DURATION OF DIET

While Keto does not really have a restricted time schedule that needs to be followed to see results. It is common for clients or followers to have week-long diets or even ten-to-fifteen-day diets followed by a two-day break. Month-long diets are also followed, but then again, they are usually accompanied by gaps in between. However, no more than two gaps are recommended by reputed Dietitians. It also must be noted that while talking about the time duration required of following Ketogenic Diet, we need to talk about the type of Ketogenic diets present currently as well. They are as follows:

o   Targeted ketogenic diet (TKD): This variant is flexible in a way that it allows the addition of extra carbohydrates when facing periods of intensive physical workout, as not to leave the recipient feeling burnt out.

o   Cyclical ketogenic diet (CKD): This diet involves periods of higher carbohydrate intake in between the ketogenic diet cycles, for example, five ketogenic days followed by two high-carbohydrate days as a cycle

o   Standard ketogenic diet (SKD): The SKD and HPKD have been used extensively. The cyclical and targeted ketogenic diets are recent additions and mostly used by bodybuilders or athletes. The SKD is the most researched and recommended, and the rest of this article will deal with SKD.

o   High-protein ketogenic diet (HPKD): This diet includes more protein and the ratio of around 60 per cent fat, 35 per cent protein and five per cent carbohydrates but as can be seen, it is still a very high fat diet.

o   (SKD): This is a very low-carbohydrate with moderate-protein and high-fat diet. It typically contains 70 per cent fat, 20 per cent protein and only 10 per cent carbohydrates.

o   A prolonged break from Ketogenic diet is not recommended as that halts the process of ketosis that had been taking place. And to get back into the running is a painstaking rendezvous point as it is with any diet you may follow.

- HOW TO REACH KETOSIS?

Ketosis, as mentioned earlier, is a process that your body goes through when it is faced with low levels of carbohydrates, so much so that it no longer has any to burn. Ketones is a by-product of this process. Thus it turns to the fat stores in your body and burns those down instead to make ketones which are used as energy stores. It doesn't just burn fat but allows you to retain your muscle's shape and firmness. Ketosis, unlike carbohydrate intake, keeps you from unnecessary round-the-clock cravings and occasional hunger pangs. It keeps you feeling full.

Ketones are basically chemicals that your liver makes when your body is in ketosis i.e. the body is burning fats instead of carbohydrates. Ketones is a type of acid that your liver releases into the bloodstream. Your muscle and tissue then utilize this acid for fuel and energy. Ketones are not the same as ketacids.

For those who aren't diabetic or pregnant ketosis normally kicks in after three or four days of low carb intake. It may also be triggered through fasting—basically, anything in the limits of fifty grams of carbohydrate intake.

- DIRTY KETO

Dirty Keto is when you eat low-quality meals in the name of Keto friendly foods while your intake is also comprising of 'bad' fats. A sole diet of Vegetable Oil, excessively processed food and fried meat intake is what can be described as bad fats. That is what brings your protein intake to twenty percent, while your carbohydrate intake is extremely low as well. This diet leads to adverse effects like sleeplessness and hair fall instead of the positive results that you wish to see, and this concept as a whole is known as Dirty Keto. Thus, it is very important to monitor your intake of food and partake in a well-balanced Keto meal plan. It should contain a combination of vegetables, proteins, fruits, and vitamins. That ensures that your body receives the necessities that it requires while you work towards a healthier lifestyle.

- MEDICAL APPLICATIONS

The Ketogenic diet was actually discovered by Russel Wilder in 1921 when he was treating epilepsy patients. Dr Russel Wilder was also the man who named it, Ketogenic Diet. For more than a decade, the diet enjoyed its position as a therapeutic diet for pediatric epilepsy and was popularly picked up all over. That is until the medicine world advanced to introduce antiepileptic agents.

Its introduction and rise to wide spread popularity as a weight-loss regime is a fairly recent concept and quite an essential one at it as well. Despite the medical advances that the medical world has experienced, obesity continues to pose a threat to the world's population. It continues to pose a health hazard as high as adult mortality as high as 2.8 million per year. Obesity is a leading factor to a majority of chronic diseases like hypertension, diabetes, and heart, all of which are almost certainly a product of poor dietary habits and an unhealthy lifestyle.

However, since it's it uses, Ketogenic diet has proven to be beneficial over a wide array of areas. Since its use, followers have claimed to reduce a person's risk of developing certain health conditions, which are not limited to cardiovascular disease, diabetes, metabolic syndrome, and even has claimed to provide better sleep and lower hair fall.

Nutritional Ketosis is beneficial for the body as it neither produces high levels of ketones which tend to become harmful and dangerous to the body. But at the same time, it also breaks down fats protecting the body from high levels of cholesterol, risk of heart disease, and high blood and sugar levels in the blood.

A small that was carried out actually once concluded that Parkinson's disease improved after twenty-eight days of following the Keto diet. So, trust me when I say the benefits to Ketogenic Diet are immense. You just have to start.

Ketogenic diets for diabetes and prediabetes
Diabetes is characterized by metabolic changes, elevated blood sugar, and decreased functioning of insulin.

A ketogenic diet can help you lose excess fat strongly linked to type 2 diabetes, metabolic syndrome, and prediabetes.

One older study showed that the ketogenic diet increased the sensitivity of insulin by a whopping 75%.

A small study in women with type 2 diabetes also found that hemoglobin A1C, an indicator of long-term blood sugar management, significantly decreased after a ketogenic diet for 90 days.

Another study of 349 individuals with type 2 diabetes showed that, over two years, those who adopted a ketogenic diet lost an average of 26.2 pounds (11.9 kg). This is a significant benefit when considering the correlation between weight and type 2 diabetes.

Also, improved blood sugar control was also experienced, and the use of some blood sugar medications decreased among participants during the study.

Other health benefits of keto
In reality, the ketogenic diet began as a method for the treatment of neurological disorders like epilepsy.

Research has now shown that diets can have benefit for a wide range of different health conditions:

• Heart disease. The ketogenic diet can help enhance risk factors like body fat, blood pressure, blood sugar, and HDL (good) cholesterol levels.

• Cancer. The diet is currently being investigated as an alternative cancer treatment, as it may help slow the tumor's growth.

• Alzheimer's disease. The keto diet will help to alleviate symptoms of Alzheimer's disease and delay its development.

• Epilepsy. Research has shown that the ketogenic diet can cause substantial reductions in seizures in epileptic children.

• Parkinson's disease. Though more study is needed, one study found that the diet helped enhance Parkinson's disease symptoms.

• Polycystic ovary syndrome. Ketogenic diet can help lower insulin levels, which can play a vital role in polycystic ovary syndrome.

• Brain injuries. Some research indicates that diet can improve the results of traumatic brain injuries.

Bear in mind, however, that research into all of these fields is far from conclusive.

Foods to avoid

Any food that is high in carbs should be limited or eliminated.

Here is a list of foods that need to be eliminated or reduced on a ketogenic diet:

fruit: all type of fruits, except small portions of berries like strawberries

sugary foods: fruit juice, smoothies, soda, cake, ice cream, candy, etc.

grains or starches: wheat-based products, pasta, rice, cereal, etc.

root vegetables and tubers: potatoes, carrots, parsnips, sweet potatoes, etc.

beans or legumes: kidney beans, lentils, peas, chickpeas, etc.

low fat or diet products: salad dressings, low-fat mayonnaise, and condiments

unhealthy fats: processed vegetable oils, mayonnaise, etc.

some condiments or sauces: honey mustard, teriyaki sauce, barbecue sauce, ketchup, etc.

sugar-free diet foods: syrups, puddings, sugar-free candies, sweeteners, desserts, etc.

alcohol: beer, wine, liquor, mixed drinks

Foods to eat

Your meals should be based around these foods:

- **meat:** ham, sausage, red meat, steak, bacon, chicken, and turkey

- **eggs:** pastured or omega-3 whole eggs

- **fatty fish:** trout, tuna, salmon, and mackerel

- **cheese:** unprocessed cheeses like goat, cream, cheddar, blue, or mozzarella

- **butter and cream:** grass-fed butter and heavy cream

- **nuts and seeds:** walnuts, flaxseeds, almonds, pumpkin seeds, chia seeds, etc.

- **avocados:** freshly made guacamole or whole avocados

- **healthy oils:** extra virgin olive oil, avocado oil, and coconut oil

- **low carb veggies:** tomatoes, onions, green veggies, peppers, etc.

- **condiments:** salt, herbs, pepper, and spices

Tips for eating out on a ketogenic diet

Many restaurant meals can be made keto-friendly.

A lot of restaurants serve some type of meat or fish-based dish. Order this and substitute any high-carb food with extra vegetables.

Egg-based meals are also a great choice, such as an egg or omelet or and bacon.

Another favorite is bun-less burgers. You may swap the fries out for vegetables as well. Add extra avocado, eggs, cheese, or bacon.

You can enjoy any type of meat at Mexican restaurants with extra guacamole, salsa, cheese, and sour cream.

For dessert, request berries with cream or mixed cheese board.

Breaking Down the Keto Diet

The keto diet is all about eating more fat and cutting carbs. Here's what the carbohydrates, protein, and fat daily breakdown look like:

• 5% of calories from carbohydrates, including non-starchy vegetables, low-carb, and small quantities of leafy greens. The keto diet excludes carb-rich foods like beans, fruits, grains, and starchy vegetables.

• 20% protein calories from protein, such as eggs, meat, and cheese.

• 75% of calories from fat, such as unprocessed nuts, butter, oils, and avocado.

According to dietitian Richelle Gomez, MS, RDN, LDN, Northwestern Medicine McHenry Hospital, the ketogenic diet is meant to burn fat by removing carbohydrates. "Your body turns carbohydrates into glucose for energy," she explains. "You switch to burning fatty acids or ketones when you cut carbs from your diet."

Ketosis is called breaking down fats for energy. It takes about three weeks of carbohydrate removal for your body to transition into ketosis.

Below are the pros and cons of the keto diet

PROS

Weight Loss

Melinda R. Ring, MD, director of the Northwestern Medicine Osher Center for Integrative Medicine, states, "There has been anecdotal evidence of people losing weight on a ketogenic diet." "People also report that they feel less hungry than on other restricted diet types."

Gomez says individuals feel less hungry because fatty foods take longer to break down in the body. Weight loss occurs not only through ketosis but also by reducing calorie consumption by eliminating food groups.

No More Low-Fat

On paper, burn fats by consuming more of them is quite enticing, which is why the diet has become popular. The keto diet allows many individuals to consume the types of high-fat foods they love, such as red meat, nuts, cheese, fatty fish, and butter, while still losing weight.

Health Benefits for Specific People

The ketogenic diet helps minimize seizures in pediatric epilepsy patients. Endurance athletes and bodybuilders also use it to scrap fat in brief timeframes. The keto diet is being examined to relieve symptoms for patients with progressive neurological conditions such as Parkinson's disease, but scientific study has not confirmed any advantages for these populations.

CONS

Difficult to Sustain

Many find the keto diet hard to adhere to because of the restrictive food restrictions.

"The keto diet can be very effective for weight loss when used within a short time followed by the adoption of healthy eating habits," says Cardiologist Kameswari Maganti, MD, Northwestern Medicine Bluhm Cardiovascular Institute." "It lends itself, unfortunately, to yo-yo dieting, which increases mortality."

It's hard to reach ketosis because it's like a light switch: either on or off. Those who track food consumption regularly are more likely to stay in ketosis. However, a blood test is the only way to know whether the body is in ketosis.

Calorie Depletion and Nutrient Deficiency

"Because the keto diet is so restricted, you are not receiving the nutrients - minerals, fibers, vitamins— that you get from fresh fruits, vegetables, legumes, and whole grains," says Dr. Ring.

As a result of these deficiencies, people also report feeling foggy and exhausted. These symptoms have been dubbed "the keto flu. Constipation is also common on the keto diet as a result of a lack of fiber.

On paper, burning fats by eating more of them is enticing.

Bad Fats in Practice

The high-fat nature of the diet may also have adverse effects on heart health. The American Heart Association recommends that saturated fat consumption should be limited to 5 to 6%. "Many people eat high amounts of saturated fats in practice, which could increase the risk of cardiovascular disease," Dr. Maganti says. "In six to eight weeks, we see an increase in lipids, or fats, in patients1 blood on the keto diet."

Renal Risk

Patients with kidney disease have a higher risk of requiring dialysis on the keto diet due to the additional ketones that their renal system has to process," says Dr. Maganti.

Some individuals often undergo dehydration on the keto diet because they eradicate glycogen, which holds water, from their bloodstream.

Food Obsession

"When you micromanage your food consumption by tracking how much you eat, It disconnects you from what your body is asking for," says Gomez. "Instead of listening to your body, you begin using outside numbers to determine what to eat."

Monitoring food closely can lead to psychological distress, such as binge eating and shame. Restriction can result in bingeing, leading to guilt, which is a continuous loop that often leads back to restriction.

Other: Approaches

For long-term weight loss, both Dr. Ring and Dr. Maganti suggest healthy approaches, including the Mediterranean diet.

"While eating a varied and balanced diet through intermittent fasting, you can still receive the benefits of ketosis," says Dr. Ring.

Gomez recommends making incremental improvements based on your health goals, . She says, "All foods fit into a healthy diet." "It is a matter of moderation and finding ways to consume the foods you love without overindulging."

WHAT IS A CHAFFLE?

A Chaffle is essentially a cheese waffle. Its two main ingredients are cheese and waffles! The flour is also replaced with eggs and not almond/nut flour as the base of the recipe and is loaded with cheese. And allow me to let you in on a little secret- they taste delicious! Chaffles mimic Waffles in shape but they are not the same thing at all. It's even called that as a play on words between waffle and cheese; how fun! Another name for Chaffle is also eggos but it's not that commonly used.

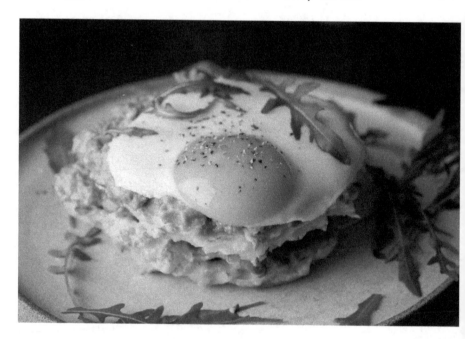

- DIFFERENCE BETWEEN CHAFFLE AND WAFFLE

You know what a basic waffle is, which is merely an amalgamation of the typical batter: eggs, flour, oil, and backing soda, served with a side of either fruits, syrup, or even a sprinkle of powdered sugar.

Now, let us introduce you to a healthier yet even tastier derivation of a waffle: The chaffle.

The essential difference between the two is that a chaffle contains more protein and less fat than a waffle.

Essentially, chaffles were invented for individuals who do not, or cannot, eat grains. Instead of using typical grains, chaffle make use of any shredded bland cheese, such as mozzarella, and combine it with egg. It also sometimes consists of a fat such as butter.

These little chaffles are pieces of heaven, and are even healthier than a waffle

- WHAT IS A KETO CHAFFLE?

A Keto Chaffle is basically a waffle made with keto-friendly ingredients. The whole word has basically been invented when a "Chaffle" recipe was uploaded on Facebook, and it just went viral. From there and then, there has been no coming back, and if may be so bold to comment, I think we have essentially crossed a point of no return.

Ever since that fated Facebook post, the possibilities and combinations that have popped up are endless- and more are on the horizon. It makes one wonder, have we truly tried them all? In all flavors and textures? Obviously, a Chaffle doesn't necessarily have to mimic the shape and texture of a waffle. The batter can simply be shaped into different molds and for different purposes. While still remaining Keto friendly, and thus body and weight friendly. What more could one possibly ask for when it comes to a recipe? It simply ticks all the boxes!

- BASIC INGREDIENT OF A CHAFFLE

Like I mentioned above, the possibilities are in a bottomless pit when it comes to experimenting your easy and beginner friendly Chaffle recipes. However, as it always is with recipes, the basic ingredients remain the same, the same concept ranks true when it comes to Chaffle recipes.

The basic ingredients of a Chaffle remain; eggs and cheese. The original formula remains a half cup of cheese and one single (egg brought to room temperature i.e.

take it out of the fridge prior to cooking) which is a tried and tested mixture that won the hearts of many.

However, some minorities have offered insights of the recipe rather eggy for the lack of a better word. Thus, the masses have tinkered and tailored and come up with recipes that were more tailored to their taste. While we may not know what your personal taste is, we sure can provide an insight that may allow you to experiment on your own. Obviously, at the end of the day, that recipe and that dish is yours. You're the one who has to cater, taste, and enjoy so please feel free to adjust it to your needs and preferences.

- CRISPY CHAFFLES

If you wish to ensure that you get the perfect crunch in your Chaffle instead of the soft bread like texture, you are definitely looking at the right place. These few tips and tricks will also help to avoid or mask the taste of egg in your Chaffles. So here we go!

The first thing you can do is simply minus the yolk in your Chaffle mixture and instead double the number of egg whites. That way the taste is quite mild and even those who get queasy at the sight of eggs can enjoy a keto friendly body friendly Chaffle whenever they like.

The second thing that you need to do is to allow your Chaffle to rest and cool down completely once it's cooked before biting into it.

- CHAFFLES AREN'T ALWAYS SWEET

Yep, you heard right. Or well-read. Either way, Chaffles don't necessarily have to be sweet. During the experimentation process of this recipes our dainty chefs have come up with Chaffles that are both; sweet and savory!

Includes the best basic Ketogenic Chaffles recipes, the savory Chaffles include basic ingredients such as jalapeno poppers and garlic parmesan. Sweet Chaffles include cinnamon churros along with pumpkin for some extra punch of flavor.

Make sure you thoroughly heat the waffle maker.

Before adding the batter, sprinkle a little cheese on the waffle iron, then a little more on top of the batter.

Make sure that the chaffle is cooked till it is golden brown. Some say that the optimal cooking time is 2-3 minutes. I prefer a 3-4-minute cooking time.

The calorie count in Chaffles will vary with the ingredients, so for it to remain keto-friendly and catered to your dietary restrictions, it must be taken care to use Keto-friendly ingredients.

- PROFESSIONAL TIPS

Here we are going to talk about a few neat tricks and tips to make the perfect Chaffle that you'll simply keep coming back to because it will just be that perfect!

1. Preheat your oven! Trust me when I say preheating is key when it comes to baking or cooking. And where Chaffles are mentioned, you want your iron to be so hot that it starts to cook the second your batter hits it.

2. Make sure you have all the ingredients as part of your prep.

3. You can melt your cream cheese in a double boiler or even a microwave. It obviously doesn't need to be

piping hot, just enough to be manageable when you stir or spread it.

4.   For savory chaffles, you can sprinkle some shredded cheese over your Chaffle iron before placing your batter. That will result in a more charred and crispier Chaffle for you to enjoy.

5.   Finely shredded is manageable as compared to thicker cut down strands.

6.   Don't restrict yourself to certain recipes, explore, experiment and create. Add cocoa powder to your batter for the perfect brownie esque Chaffles, or Oreos if that is more your cup of tea.

7.   You'll know your Chaffle is done when there is no steam coming out of the Chaffle maker anymore.

Chaffles can be gluten-free, low carb, easy to make and readily made so they can be yours go to snack anywhere, anytime.

• TOOLS REQUIREMENT

Each recipe is unique on its own. But certain recipes require basic tools that you probably have around the house as well. Just to be on the safe side we will list all of those which may be useful in this recipe.

• A spatula; to ensure you don't waste any of the batter.

• A measuring bowl; to ensure you use the correct amount of ingredients for the perfect balance of flavor and the right amount for the people you wish to make it for

• Mixing Bowl; to combine all the ingredients in.

• Handheld/Countertop Beaters; for the perfect consistency of a batter, all the ingredients need to be very well combined, for which a spatula mix would be rendered incomplete. Thus for top-notch batter you require a beater.

• Waffle Iron; while this isn't a necessity if you wish for crisp sides and the proper round waffle shape, the iron is the only way to achieve it.

• Pan; Chaffle can be made in a pancake manner on a pan.

• Oven; if you wish to make Chaffle buns you need to bake the batter in a preheated oven.

- Baking Tray; an oven-friendly tray to place your batter on.

- Baking sheet; to line the baking tray with so the batter doesn't stick to the pan and is easily removed

- Waffle irons are available in different sizes for you to get the perfect crunch and size. So explore and invest in which you think suits you best!

- CAN YOU MAKE CHAFFLES WITHOUT A WAFFLE MAKER?

While you can make chaffles without a waffle maker, the only drawback to it is that you won't get those crunchy sides anymore. If you can live without those, by all means there remains no need to invest in a Waffle Maker. You will basically be making these the same way you make keto pancakes. Just instead of a Waffle iron, pour or spread your batter on a hot non-stick pack and allow it to cook till it turns golden brown. Flip with a spatula and repeat until desired color and texture appears.

- HOW TO SERVE CHAFFLES?
  - Oh, oh the possibilities of having and serving a Chaffle are truly endless! They basically are solely

dependent on type of Chaffle you made; savory or sweet. But let's give you some over the top ideas for either.

- For some sweet Chaffles, simply drizzle some maple syrup. For some Keto-friendly options go for sugar free jams and syrups. The world is your oyster my friend!
- Add melted cheese as toppings!
- Make a Chaffle sandwich! Pile on some lettuce, tomatoes, fresh vegetables and some sausages and make yourself a delish sandwich!
- Serve with fresh fruit like strawberries or blueberries- healthy and yum!
- Top with spicy jalapenos and olives.
- Simply spread some butter and dig in
- Experiment! Mix and match till you find your perfect mouthful!

- STORING YOUR CHAFFLES

Storing your chaffles is easy. All you need is an air tight container and you're good to go. Store your chaffles in that and lock it in the fridge. And whenever you open that container up, the chaffles will be as good as ever.

- CAN YOU FREEZE YOUR CHAFFLES?

Yes! You can freeze your chaffles! How great is that. All you require is parchment paper and a tray. Or you can place them with parchment papers in between in a storage container and pop them in the freezer. Freezer bags of all shapes and sizes may be used as well and are more preferred as they are more convenient and occupy less space in your freezer.

- HOW TO REHEAT YOUR CHAFFLES

After taking your chaffles out of the freezer or fridge, the only thing to do before digging in is reheating them. For that you can basically use anything. You can heat them in your oven at 360F degrees, pop it over in a skillet and heat it over the fire. Or simply and my way of heating; is tossing them in a toaster with the lightest spread of butter and enjoying the perfect Chaffle without the fuss of even making it.

AFTERMATH OF CHAFFLE MAKING

And once all the fuss is over, the dreaded dishes are to be tackled. It's a conundrum every time isn't it? When the food that has been inhaled and ingested, the cute plates in which you so painstakingly plated, maybe even took a photo or two to post on the gram. And now all that is left are empty plates, and the awaiting sink.

- CLEANING THE CHAFFLE MAKER

It is necessary that you establish a routine when it comes to cleaning your waffle irons or machines. The trick is to ensure they are neither too hot that you harm yourself, but you also don't put it away for so long that you eventually forget about it entirely- that's a horrifying site, I assure you.

If you had used a waffle maker, like I said, allow it to cool down first before you actually start the cleaning process. Then use a damp dishcloth or kitchen towel to scoop up or wipe off any crumbs or drips around the grid plates. Make sure to get in all the nooks and crannies! The cloth will also absorb any excess oil or butter.

A neat trick to clean the stubborn little burnt batter from your grid plates is to pour in a few drops of cooking oil over those corners. Allow it to sit and absorb and ensure that the hardened batter softens. Then use the cloth to completely wipe the mess off of your Chaffle maker.

Certain Chaffle makers are now available with removable cooking plates. Those can be easily scooped up, rinsed, and washed with warm washing liquid as well. After that, it's up to you whether you air dries them or use a cloth to wipe off any moisture.

Use a damp cloth or sponge to clear out the exterior of your machine and voila, the kitchen appliance is good as new!

Obviously, had you chosen to cook your chaffles a different way, perhaps a non-stick pan. That appliance would require to be cleaned and stored in a different manner. For a non-stick pan, ensure that it does not require to be soaked so any burnt batter spots may be softened and removed. You must be careful not to put any pressure on the pan as to not damage the non-stick layer. Use a sponge and warm water to gently but effectively clean the pan. And allow it to air dry before you store it.

- TIPS FOR WAFFLE MAKER MAINTENANCE

For those of us who are frequent Chaffle munchers, we know that at times oil gathers in the iron grid. And my God, can those stains be annoying. For those, take a chopstick or a long toothpick and warp a damp cloth or a kitchen towel around the pointy end of it. Moisten that tip with vinegar of any kind and use that to wipe away any residue or oil droplets from your grid. And don't forget to thank me later!

Although this goes without saying but still is quite important, so I will start with this. Always read your instruction manuals! The tiny booklet of user manual with directions is quite honestly your little book of answers. So always make sure that you have gone through when you buy a Chaffle Iron, or any kitchen appliance for that matter.

The next tip seems rather obvious as well, but I'll just go ahead reinstate it as well. Never submerge an electric waffler iron in the water. It's neither good for the appliance and could be a health hazard as well.

With the obvious do's and don'ts out of the way, let me indulge you in some habits I have adopted to keep my Waffle iron top-notch even after all these years of use!

Considering you own a non-stick Waffle maker, you must know that it only needs a light coating of cooking oil before use, and that too for a complete batch. A fresh coating is not required for every individual Chaffle. I prefer using a pastry brush to layer that coat of oil as it remains gentle. Also, arsenal oil tends to leave a sticky residue behind on a non-stick so it's best to choose wisely.

If while removing your cooked Chaffle, it seems stuck at some point, never use sharp metal tools to chip off the stuck batter. All that will accomplish is maybe a scratch on the surface. And it will most likely create a future problem while not even solving the one at hand.

However, under the circumstance that your Chaffle does begin to stick, just ensure that you're using an ample amount of oil to grease your Chaffle. And if you are check if the amount of butter you've used is correct or not. The higher ratio of butter, the less chance there is that your Chaffle will stick to the surface.

That about it about Chaffles, I hope it answered every question you might have had- or didn't have!